Maximum Style Editorial Staff

Managing Editor: **Jack Croft**

Writers: **Perry Garfinkel, Brian Chichester, Donna Raskin**

Assistant Research Manager: **Jane Unger Hahn**

Lead Researcher: **Tanya H. Bartlett**

Editorial Researchers: **Carol J. Gilmore, Nanci Kulig, Sally A. Reith, Jennifer Schaeffer, Staci Ann Sander**

Copy Editors: **Amy K. Kovalski, David R. Umla**

Series Art Director: **Charles Beasley**

Series Designer: **John Herr**

Book Designer: **Thomas P. Aczel**

Cover Designer: **Charles Beasley**

Cover Photographer: **Walter Smith**

Illustrators: **Thomas P. Aczel, Mark Matcho**

Layout Artist: **Mary Brundage**

Manufacturing Coordinator: **Melinda B. Rizzo**

Office Manager: **Roberta Mulliner**

Office Staff: **Julie Kehs, Mary Lou Stephen**

Rodale Health and Fitness Books

Vice-President and Editorial Director: **Debora T. Yost**

Executive Editor: **Neil Wertheimer**

Design and Production Director: **Michael Ward**

Research Manager: **Ann Gossy Yermish**

Copy Manager: **Lisa D. Andruscavage**

Studio Manager: **Stefano Carbini**

Book Manufacturing Director: **Helen Clogston**

Photo Credits

All photographs by **Mitch Mandel** except those listed below.

Page 146: **Bill Luster**

Page 148: **CBS News**

Page 150: **Mark Allan**

Page 152: **Four Seasons/Regent Hotels and Resorts**

Page 154: **World Championship Wrestling**

Page 160: **FPG**

Page 161: **JFK Library**

Page 162: **Frank Driggs Collection**

Page 163: **FPG**

Contents

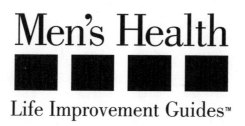

Men's Health

Life Improvement Guides™

Maximum Style

Look Sharp and Feel Confident in Every Situation

by Perry Garfinkel, Brian Chichester, and the Editors of **Men'sHealth** Books

Reviewed by Ken Karpinski of Sterling, Virginia, image consultant to Fortune 500 companies, the U.S. Military, and numerous corporate executives, and author of *Red Socks Don't Work*

Rodale Press, Inc.
Emmaus, Pennsylvania

Copyright © 1997 by Rodale Press, Inc.

Cover photograph copyright © 1997 by Walter Smith
Illustrations copyright © 1997 by Mark Matcho

Printed in the United States of America on acid-free ∞, recycled paper ♻

Other titles in the *Men's Health Life Improvement Guides* series:

Fight Fat	*Stress Blasters*
Food Smart	*Stronger Faster*
Powerfully Fit	*Symptom Solver*
Sex Secrets	

Library of Congress Cataloging-in-Publication Data

Garfinkel, Perry.
    Maximum style : look sharp and feel confident in every situation / by Perry Garfinkel, Brian Chichester, and the editors of Men's Health Books.
       p. c.m. — (Men's health life improvement guides)
    Includes index.
    ISBN 0–87596–379–X paperback
    1. Men's clothing. 2. Grooming for men. 3. Men—Life skills guides. I. Chichester, Brian. II. Men's Health Books. III. Title. IV. Series.
    TT617.G37 1997
    646'.32—dc21
                                                         97–3799

Distributed in the book trade by St. Martin's Press

2 4 6 8 10 9 7 5 3 1   paperback

OUR PURPOSE

*"We inspire and enable people to improve
their lives and the world around them."*

Part Four
Always in Style

Part Five
Real-Life Scenarios

Introduction

The Secret to True Style

Talk to enough style mavens—as we did for this book—and you can't help but come away shaking your head. If your quest is to discover the secret to true personal style, you'll find plenty of answers. More than you bargained for, in fact. Here are some that you'll find in the pages that follow.

- "If there is one article of clothing that defines a man, it is his pants. They are the universal symbol of masculinity."
- "Your shirt defines who you are more than any other item," says Mark Weber, vice-chairman of Phillips–Van Heusen Corporation in New York City, the country's largest shirt maker, and author of *Dress Casually for Success... for Men.*
- "When it comes to style, underwear may very well be the real window to the soul," says Ross E. Goldstein, Ph.D., a psychologist and president of Generation Insights, a consulting company in San Francisco. "They're one of the last bastions of self-expression."
- "Shoes can often be the most obvious sign of a man's sense of style and social position," says Alan Flusser, a New York City menswear designer and author of *Style and the Man.*

It got to be an inside joke around here as we wrote this book: Somehow, every "expert" we talked with gave a different answer for what was the single most important component to style. Your tie. Your sport coat. Your suit. Your jewelry. Then there were the experts who looked beyond clothing. So mix in the way that you comb your hair, whether you grow a beard, how you care for your nails, and what kind of aftershave or cologne you wear. And then, just for good measure, toss in the intangibles: how you react under pressure, whether you convey confidence, whether you merely walk into a room or make an entrance. And pretty soon, you feel like tossing in the towel because it seems like *everything* is the most important thing in terms of style.

And that, my friends, is precisely the point.

Everything is important. When you're talking about creating your own personal style, each of the seemingly insignificant little decisions that you make about how you look, dress, and conduct yourself makes a difference. The key is to see the big picture—decide who you are and how you want others to see you—and then put all the elements together in a style that is uniquely your own.

Sound tough? Well, with the book that you're holding in your hands, it just got a whole lot easier.

Maximum Style is unlike any other fashion and grooming book that you'll find because we at *Men's Health* Books believe that style is an individual matter. There is no one look that fits all. And most of the sins against style committed by men—leisure suits and Nehru jackets come to mind—happened because too many guys fell for the old trick of letting someone else tell them what looked good. I don't know about you, but when I look around the office here, I don't see many guys who look like they stepped out of a Madison Avenue ad campaign or a Hollywood set.

But I do see more than a few men of true style. Men of passion and conviction. Men who dress and act confidently, whether it's Casual Friday at the office or a formal banquet at a posh ballroom. Men not susceptible to the vagaries of high fashion. Men with poise, humor, character. These are the kind of men that we admire. This is the kind of man that you can be.

Maximum Style can help. Think of it as your personal image consultant. Use the information that we've culled from some of the leading style experts to make sure that the man others see is the man you want to be.

Jack Croft

Jack Croft
Managing Editor, *Men's Health* Books

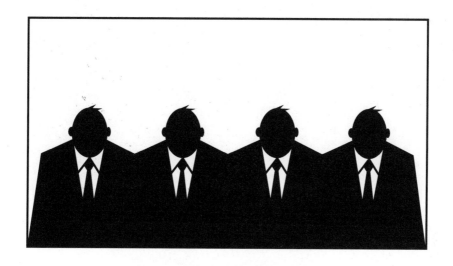

Part One

Elements of Style

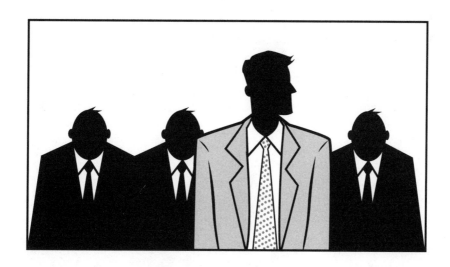

A Man of Style

What It All Means

"He has style."

Admit it: You've always wanted people to say that about you. And yet, when you try to define style, you inevitably stumble. For most of us, the concept of style remains elusive and ambiguous, a vague mix of clothes and possessions, hair and voice, persona and presence.

Because we can't exactly pin it down, we often put it down. How many times have you heard—or said yourself—that something represented the "triumph of style over substance," as though the two concepts were mutually exclusive. They're not. This is the first fundamental truth about maximum style: Unless you're a man of substance, you'll never acquire style.

The Substance of Style

To define what precisely it means to have maximum style, we talked to scores of experts. Fashion psychologists, trend forecasters, image consultants, designers, manufacturers, marketers, celebrities, regular guys, and, yes, even runway commentators and their pouty models. We found that while style indeed is a many-splendored (and a highly subjective and capricious) thing, there were solid underlying themes.

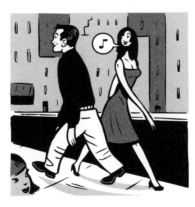

Style, for example, clearly includes a sharp sense of dress. What you wear says an enormous amount about who you are, what you stand for, how you live. That's obvious.

But what makes for stylish dress isn't so clear. And it doesn't mean expensive. It doesn't mean current. It doesn't mean outlandish. Dressing well falls in that well-worn category of things that you can't define, but you know it when you see it.

Style also means smart grooming. The subtleties of your hair, your fingernails, your breath, and your skin all add up to making an important statement about how you value your appearance.

But more than anything else, style is about demeanor. A man of style carries himself with dignity, with strength, with purpose, with confidence. These are not visual qualities, and yet you see them instantly in a man. It is how he carries his head, shakes hands, or uses eye contact; it is how he smiles or laughs; it is how he fits into any situation so naturally, so quickly.

Ultimately, style is about being yourself. It is about knowing exactly who you are and then crafting a look that projects that, without compromise or bending to the winds of fashion or peer pressure. This is the second fundamental truth about style.

"When you talk about style, I think of someone who's not a follower. Someone who's self-assured, comfortable with himself, and confident enough to know that he creates his own style. That's what people admire," says Jeff Livingston, Ph.D., past director of the National Association of Business Consultants in Raleigh, North Carolina, and an information analyst for Cisco Systems in Research Triangle Park, North Carolina.

"When you say, 'He has style,' I would reserve that for the person who conducts himself appropriately," suggests Michael R. Losey, president and chief executive officer of the Society for Human Resource Management, a professional organization in Alexandria, Virginia. "In other words, someone who's honest, straightforward, and credible. Someone who has demonstrated that he's bright and informed and is balanced in his life."

In short, it sounds like the stuff that you were taught as a kid but too easily forget as an adult.

Do Clothes Make the Man?

How you dress is certainly part of the style equation. But it's not—as many mistakenly seem to think—the whole thing.

"To me, style is a person who understands what he can wear and how to put it together in a way that no one else can," states Marvin Pieland, manager and clothing consultant for Saks Fifth Avenue Club for Men in New York City. "It's not necessarily requiring a designer name to validate your appearance. It's being able to create your own image in a way that draws attention to your better features without making you look ridiculous."

You might think that stylish men spend a lot of money to look and act that way. And obviously, some do. Some buy expensive designer clothes. Some go to charm school. Some take voice lessons and hire image consultants. But here's the third fundamental truth about maximum style: Like love, money can't buy it.

"You don't have to spend a lot to have style; you simply do not," affirms Ken Karpinski of Sterling, Virginia, image consultant to Fortune 500 companies, the U.S. military, and numerous corporate executives, and author of *Red Socks Don't Work*.

Style's Most Wanted

What are the characteristics of a stylish man? When Levi Strauss prepared to launch its Slates menswear line in 1996, the jeans giant hired Ross E. Goldstein, Ph.D., a psychologist and president of Generation Insights, a consulting company in San Francisco, to find out. According to Dr. Goldstein's survey of 522 randomly selected American men, here's what he found were the most sought-after traits of a successful image and how they rated.

Confidence	60%
Keeping cool under pressure	51%
Understanding and caring	49%
Being smart	41%
Being practical and realistic	37%
Competitiveness	36%
Being flexible and accommodating	34%
Aggressiveness	23%
Cautiousness	21%
Being good-looking	6%

"Of all the things that have to do with creating an image, expensive clothing and accessories are almost always one of the last factors," Karpinski says. "In fact, in today's casual workforce, clothing in many ways is less important than ever."

The clothes you do buy, casual or not, don't have to cost a mint, either. Even frugal finds can look dashing. How? If you know what to look for, you can buy good-quality clothes on sale or at discount merchandisers. Or you can spruce up your wardrobe with pricey accessories. Or mix and match apparel, for example, to accentuate a more expensive jacket and tie and de-emphasize that $30 oxford-knit shirt.

"Manufacturers have made style available to everyone these days," says fashion expert Leon Hall of New York City, who is creative director for International Apparel Mart in Dallas, spokesperson for The Fashion Association, and a frequent fashion commentator and trend forecaster.

Hall cites the move by lower-end retailers, such as Kmart, to upscale their clothing lines, and of mid-level outfits, like JCPenney and Levi Strauss—with their successful Dockers franchise—as style opportunities that have opened doors for the less affluent.

"With an eye as trained as mine, of course, I can usually tell who made what from across the room; but that's how I make my living," Hall says. "Many times, though, I want to save money, too. I have a pair of great shoes from Sears, for example, and I love them. Clothes that look the best don't always cost the most."

Fashion versus Style

For the record, there's a difference between fashion and style. Fashion is temporal. Fleeting. It changes with the seasons, and, like David Bowie, you see it again and again in new incarnations. According to Roland Barthes, author of the groundbreaking 1967 book *The Fashion System*, fashion reaches its extremes every 100 years, deviating from the "norm" about every 50.

"Fashion is so accurately the reflection of the society who wears it," says David Wolfe, creative director and chief trend forecaster at The Doneger Group, a buying house and fashion forecasting firm in New York City. Look at the buttoned-down, dark days of the Puritans, the urbane overcoat of the frumpish 1850s, the refined elegance of the turn of the century, and the rebellious hippie look popular in the 1960s. Each reflected the era's zeitgeist and, more often than not, according to Wolfe, the goings-on politically, religiously, and sociologically.

Style, on the other hand, is less mercurial and more enduring. "Some people think that the core of the matter, style, is what's important; but you can't deny that others judge you based on whether you look 'in' or 'out' with what's in vogue," says Kirt Mancuso, marketing services manager for Florsheim, a footwear manufacturer in Chicago.

If they had to choose, most experts come down on the side of style, not fashion. Keeping up with the fickle finger of fashion isn't for the fainthearted. First, it's an exercise in futility, because what you're wearing now will differ from what's hot next fall. Moreover, it's impractical. Who wants to pay $700 for a new designer Nehru jacket when you threw your old, tattered one out 15 years ago?

"It's like Shakespeare said when he wrote, 'All the world's a stage,' " says image consultant Louise Elerding, president of the Association of Image Consultants International and owner of The Color Studio in Glendale, California. "We are all actors, and we're wearing our costumes every day. If you have to be cutting-edge, it's probably because it's expected in your profession or lifestyle. Most people don't fall into that category."

What Matters Most

This book teems with practical advice from the experts about all things style. We'll discuss in detail how to dress and groom yourself to put forth the exact persona that you wish to convey. Moreover, we'll show you ways to carry yourself with confidence and strength. But to start, we'll leave you with two simple, yet all-encompassing, suggestions.

1. Observe thyself. The two faces of style—yours and society's—must blend harmoniously, and the only way that they're going to do that is through diligence on your part.

"Everything we do, everything we say, everything we wear conveys something about us," Karpinski says. "Your accoutrements, your pen, your shoes, the car you're driving. If a guy is driving a lime green Corvair, he's telling you something about his personality on a certain level."

Continually evaluate yourself by asking, "What is this saying about me? Is this the message that I want to convey? Am I comfortable with this message? Can I improve or alter it?" Apply these questions to everything: your wardrobe, your car, your shoes, socks, haircut, speaking voice, sense of humor, and so on. Rarely do we embark on such self-discovery unprompted, but when we do, it's well worth the effort.

2. Equip thyself. This weekend, pull your closet apart and take inventory. And while you're at it, give all your shirts, pants, and shoes a good close-up inspection while everything's lying on your bed.

"There's a lot of work to be done," Elerding says.

Look for frayed cuffs, yellowed necklines, ring-around-the-collar, spots and stains, rips and tears, fabric that's worn too thin, scuff marks on your shoes, breaking shoelaces, food stains on ties, and the like. Also get a feel for your wardrobe in the big picture: Do you have too many casual clothes? Too many white shirts? Too many paisley ties? No brown shoes? Do you need a blazer or new suit? A tux of your own?

The Cost of Higher Education

If polishing your image is truly important, consider calling on a professional consultant to get some formal training. All told, it's not a big expense, and it's money invested in yourself and your future.

"It's a good solid education that you can use for the rest of your life," says Louise Elerding of the Association of Image Consultants International and The Color Studio. Here's what you'd be looking to pay.

- $50 for self-help reference books on image, wardrobe, and etiquette. You keep these.
- $250 to $300 for a consultation that should include getting your colors done, a review and evaluation of your wardrobe, clarification of your goals and style considerations, body proportion measurements, head-to-toe assessment, lifestyle assessment, and a review of your own observations.

"I want to know your lifestyle, whether you're married or single, employed or unemployed, boss or employee, your personal goals, your goals within the company—everything," says image consultant and makeup artist Princess Jenkins, owner of Majestic Images International, an image consulting firm in New York City. "Details are important."

- $1,000 for wardrobe adjustments, if necessary.
- $150 for seminars and classes at your community college on etiquette, public speaking, voice training, or whatever subject you'd like to improve upon.

Grand total? About $1,500 for information and education that could change your life.

Defining Yourself

How to Be a Man of Substance

Set aside thoughts of clothing, grooming, and strutting for a moment. Before all that come some deeper, harder lessons.

You see, a true man of style is someone who is true to himself. Someone who has a clear conception of who he is and what he wants to accomplish in life and whose actions and choices are governed by that knowledge. So before you can even attempt to remake or refine your wardrobe, appearance, or image—which is what this book is primarily about—you must first answer those deep, fundamental questions about yourself.

"People who have and know their values and who don't neglect their values are, by definition, the most compelling and attractive individuals in our society," says Dr. Ross E. Goldstein of Generation Insights. "You have to be comfortable with yourself and any decision that you make. There are lots of ways of conveying power and self-confidence, but these are among the most powerful. People who know and accept themselves inherently have more personal style."

What You Value

You are a unique creation within the entire history of time. And we're not just talking about DNA and technical, scientific distinctions. No one before you were born was you, and no one after you die will be you. The question, then, is, What are you going to be while you're here? Too often, we get so swept up in the swift currents of our daily lives—our jobs, families, obliga-

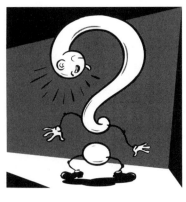

tions—that we pay no attention to where it is that those currents are carrying us.

"It's important when you're navigating job and career choices, in particular, to know and stick strongly to your deep, personal feelings," says sociologist Jan Yager, Ph.D., of Stamford, Connecticut, author of *Making Your Office Work for You* and numerous other books for business professionals.

"These are your ethics. These are your values and principles. If they're not given the emphasis that they deserve, it'll catch up to you," Dr. Yager says.

Think about the men you admire. The men whose style you would most like to emulate. They may be ruggedly good-looking. They may have impeccable taste in clothing and a certain elegance and dignity in the way that they carry themselves. But there almost certainly is something deeper, more profound, about them that you relate to. A sense of self. A code by which they live, much like the mythological heroes of the Old West. Defining that code, that set of values by which you will live, is essential to defining your personal style.

"There still isn't enough concern about values in this country," Dr. Yager says. "It's not given the emphasis that it deserves."

Here are some strategies to help you live by your own code.

Go back to your childhood. When Ebeneezer Scrooge embarked on his transforming journey of self-discovery in Charles Dickens's classic, *A Christmas Carol*, he started with his childhood, remembering his dreams, aspirations, and the one true love of his life. So should you.

"A lot of it goes back to your early years. What were you good at? What did you enjoy most? What came naturally to you? What did you want to be when you were a child?" Dr. Yager says. Most of us have plenty of signs that we've forgotten or have been conditioned to ignore. Maybe you're a frustrated computer programmer who has always loved to draw. There's a good chance that that repressed artist is the real you.

Find the genius within. Another sign of the real you lies with your passions, says writer, lecturer, and international consultant Ann McGee-Cooper, Ed.D., author of *You Don't Have to Go Home from Work Exhausted* and *Building Brain Power*.

"I've spent my life studying genius, and I really believe that we all have genius within us. Most of us hide it from ourselves, which is why most of us lead ordinary lives," Dr. McGee-Cooper says. "Whatever delights or interests you is a signal that that's what appeals to you. Your brain has a high response to that activity, so it's likely that that's where some of your genius lies."

See a pro. Consider talking to a career counselor to launch your adventure of self-discovery. It's his job to help people who are questioning their motivations and aspirations.

Ask for an evaluation. In lieu of seeing a pro, ask some trusted friends, mentors, and confidants to write down exactly how they perceive you. Ask them to describe your personality, your strengths, your weaknesses, your ideal job. The key is feedback.

Put yourself to the test. Your local community college job-placement office may offer a battery of tests that will gauge your ideal job tendencies and personality type. It's worth checking out.

Find inspiration in others. It's comforting to know that philosophers, wise men, writers, scholars, and psychologists have been wrestling for years with the importance of man knowing himself. "Thinking about this and developing this type of knowledge is one of the most important things that anyone can do,"

To the Death

Understanding one simple fact may help transform your life, says Bernie Siegel, M.D., former clinical professor of surgery at Yale University School of Medicine, pioneer in mind-body medicine, and author of *Love, Medicine, and Miracles*; *How to Live between Office Visits*; and *Peace, Love, and Healing*.

"You're going to die," Dr. Siegel says. "You only have a limited time here, so go live your life. If you get busy enough fixing your world and your relationships and making life work, you'll get so involved in activities of love that you may forget that you're supposed to get tired and old and die."

To get the same perspective-building effect without the danger of a near-death experience, Dr. Siegel suggests the following exercise: Write your own death certificate.

"Your name's on it. What age do you die? What of?" he says. "On my own, I die at 98 falling off my roof with my family yelling, 'You shouldn't be up there at your age.' "

Princess Jenkins of Majestic Images International says. "Don't be afraid to look inside and let what you see out."

Strike a brain balance. The left side of the brain is thought to govern logic and reasoning, while the right side is geared toward creativity and innovation. Dr. McGee-Cooper suggests paying close attention to what you're hardwired for and then making a conscious effort to exercise the underworked half.

"The key is focusing on what side is active and when. Most of us cycle through right- and left-brain preference every 90 minutes. By working with your cycle, you'll maximize your energy and productiveness," she says. By knowing your preference and working the subordinate side of your personality, you'll maximize your potential.

Cultivating Confidence

How to Develop Poise and Presence

Ask any image consultant worth his fancy fountain pen and he'll tell you that confidence is a cornerstone to style. It doesn't matter what fabric hangs from your shoulders, or if your shoes are so shiny that they signal distant planes. If you don't believe in yourself, your accoutrements are superfluous.

"A power suit will never save you if you're coming off as a Milquetoast," says image consultant Ken Karpinski.

Confidence is often mistakenly confused with arrogance, particularly in the highly competitive corporate world. We're not saying that you have to be an overbearing jerk to be successful. Confidence can—and often should—be quiet, not loud. You don't have to be Muhammad Ali, telling the world that you are the greatest. Ali, after all, was one of the true originals of this century. He could get away with it because he *was* Ali. Just look at how phony and pathetic most other athletes come across when they mimic his act.

True confidence comes from knowing who you are and what you're capable of doing. And it can be conveyed in many ways—most of them without uttering a word.

"Confidence is many things to many people, but you can't go wrong knowing the basics: good posture, a firm handshake, excellent eye contact, intellect, a sense of humor, and a pleasant speaking voice," says Louise

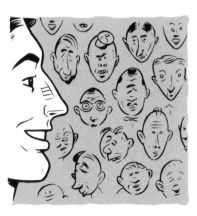

Elerding of the Association of Image Consultants International and The Color Studio.

Being Self-Assured

Here's how to radiate the confidence you need for maximum style.

Play the part. We don't always feel confident. Sure, we'd all love to be James Bond, calmly in control of every situation with a beautiful woman in one hand and a martini in the other. But there is a very practical lesson that each of us can learn from those Bond movies: Confidence, to some degree, is acting, says David Wolfe of The Doneger Group.

"In some ways you must play the part. You might feel nervous on the inside, but that's natural," Wolfe says. "Remember that it's what's showing on the outside that other people see, and you're judged by that performance even if it doesn't jive with what's going on in your head."

Dress for success. Since prehistoric times, what a man wore signified his station in life. For a caveman chieftain, the bigger the bone in his bearskin suit, the more powerful he was. This custom persists today and is deeply ingrained in our social psyche: the policeman's uniform, the priest's collar, the doctor's scrubs. Each conjures respect at face value.

Realize, then, that what you wear does influence others and can make you appear more in control. "In tennis, if you show up in traditional whites, people think that you can play regardless of your skill," Karpinski says. "If you're in grubby shorts, sneakers, and a T-shirt, you have to prove your skill."

Shake on it. You can literally have confidence at your fingertips. Handshakes are one of the first and most important impressions that we make, and the other person will conjure up all sorts of unflattering images of you if you give him a fistful of gelatin when you meet.

"The handshake tells you right away whether a man is powerful. Whether he's friendly and outgoing, or shy and timid," says Wolfe. To convey confidence, make sure that the webbing between your thumb and index finger meets his. Grasp his whole hand. Use firm pressure but don't crush his paw into hamburger, or the image he'll have of you will be Herman Munster.

Look confident. When it comes to being self-assured, the eyes have it. "Eyes are of primary importance," says Elerding. Here are her tips for poised peepers.

- Keep eye contact. Especially when you're meeting someone for the first time. Being shifty-eyed makes you look like you're trying to hide something.
- Don't wear tinted glasses indoors. "There's a perception that you're hiding something," Elerding says. "You and your glasses want to be seen as open and clear." Ditto for wearing sunglasses indoors, no matter how hungover you might be. There is one exception: Jack Nicholson.
- Don't stare. Prolonged eye contact means that you want someone dead or in bed. Make sure to keep eye contact with a tempo and blink or nod frequently to show that you're interested and paying attention. Using your eyes like a period at the end of a sentence gives your eye contact a cadence, Elerding says. "It's almost like your eyes and the words are moving to a beat."

Speak with authority. Voice projection speaks volumes about your self-assurance. Ever hear a cop whisper when he's giving you a ticket? Train yourself to speak boldly, with a

well-projected but pleasant voice. Don't boom—you'll sound overbearing. But speak with conviction. Practice on a tape recorder, lowering your voice an octave or two, no matter how painful it is to hear yourself on tape.

Getting in the Flow

Researchers have documented the ultimate feeling of confidence. It's a psychological state called flow, when athletes and others find themselves so engrossed in what they're doing that they enter an almost meditative state of bliss.

Researchers at the University of Queensland in Australia studied flow state in 28 elite-level athletes in seven sports and found some interesting correlations. Here are what they found to be the four most common elements of the flow experience.

1. Total enjoyment. Ninety-six percent of the athletes studied said that they were acutely aware of completely enjoying what they were doing. One rower described his mental state while rowing as "a little bit of magic."

2. Being one with the action. It sounds like a line from the old *Kung Fu* television series, but 86 percent of the athletes surveyed felt as if they and their actions were one with their surroundings.

3. Control without effort. Eighty-two percent of the athletes reached a state where they felt in complete control of what they were doing. Paradoxically, they weren't worried about attaining or maintaining control, nor were they actively trying to. It just happened. A field hockey player described it as "a feeling of absolute calm."

4. Laser focus. Eighty-two percent of the athletes studied said that they narrowed their concentration in flow state so that they were focused on just one thing: the task at hand. Nothing else mattered. Said a rugby player, you "shut out the crowd of 60,000 . . . you come down to a microworld down there, and there's only yourself."

Being Your Own Man

How to Assert Your Individuality

There's a story of an old Zen master who would dramatically hold up one finger every time someone asked him for the secret to enlightenment.

One day, the master learned that his closest assistant was answering questions about enlightenment the same way, so he dragged the young monk into his chambers and cut off his assistant's offending finger.

The master turned to the monk and asked, "Now then, what is the secret to enlightenment?"

The young assistant went to raise his finger, as he had done before, but it wasn't there. He smiled, for in that instant, he realized that enlightenment means knowing how to be yourself.

I, Me, Mine

When we talk about stylish men, it's almost always those who have a strong sense of who they are. It's more than just dressing well or showing good manners. Being your own man comes from deep within. It's not a designer label, a hairstyle, or a cologne. It's not an external affectation, like a cigar, a derby, or chain belt.

"Being your own man is an attitude. It's a sense of self, an expression of your soul," says David Wolfe of The Doneger Group. "Most men don't give this much thought; they seem to have more interesting things to do. Instead,

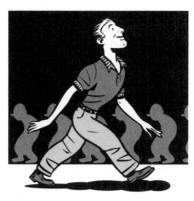

they'll follow someone else's lead."

We face tremendous pressure—some subtle, some blatantly obvious—to conform. But even in the most buttoned-down, rigid settings, there is room for you to be your own man. Here are some ways to not only maintain your individuality but also assert it.

Do what gives you pleasure. To be your own man means not letting others dictate how you act, what you wear, or where you spend your time. A man of style knows the fads and generally ignores them. If he likes tea more than coffee, then he orders tea when everyone else orders cappuccino.

He also doesn't take up tennis because the boss loves to play, or drink microbrew beer to impress his buddies. Instead, he does what he likes, unabashedly, whether it be cooking, hang gliding, volunteering at the local library, or collecting pottery.

Surround yourself with people you like. Do you think that the janitor is a great guy? Then be his friend—with pride. In the civilized world there is no caste system. Today, a man true to himself doesn't let social conventions or peer pressure choose his acquaintances or friends. The truly wise man has friends of many ages, backgrounds, educations, and beliefs. The commonality is that they all spark his mind or soul in some way that he values.

Don't mistake contrariness for uniqueness. Merely having the opposite opinion doesn't make you an individual. Good or bad, these days it is almost trendy to be cynical, to challenge all authority, to question everything, and to tear people and institutions down. Sometimes it is valid and even fun to do, a type of mental gymnastics; sometimes it's just obnoxious. The bottom line is this: A man with positive energy is a greater force than a man with negative energy. Want to be your own man? Make the world a better place not just by tearing down the bad but by offering some good, both in words and actions.

Be modest. Being your own man often means that you have hobbies, achievements, even friends that are unique. You should be proud of this. But don't brag. Nothing will make you seem more common than touting all the things that you did over the weekend. A man of style carries himself with dignity and humility; he does what he does not to impress others but to make himself happy.

Don't be mucho macho. "Confident individuals are not hampered by a masculine image anymore," says Leon Hall of International Apparel Mart and The Fashion Association. This extends from appearance (wearing an earring or shorts, for example) to expressing emotions (letting a tear drop when Ingrid Bergman gets on the plane, leaving Humphrey Bogart behind in *Casablanca*) to being one of the guys (telling your pals to can it when they start describing what they would like to do to that new "babe" in accounting).

Looking Unique

Much of this book is about how to craft a look that matches your personality. Here are a couple of ideas to start with.

Take care with what you wear. Even if you're forced to wear polyester to work or to don a pair of nondescript overalls, it doesn't mean that you're forced to turn a blind eye to your wardrobe. Everything you wear says something about your style and personality, if not just your mood for the day.

"I firmly believe that there's a lumberjack in Oregon today who is discussing, or at least thinking about, whether he should wear plaid or denim," says Hall. "Just because you may be

---

Uniform Individuals

In another life, in another world, in another universe, Jim Schneck might have boldly gone where no man has gone before. Instead, he spends his time closer to home, in his community, as chief of the Emmaus Ambulance Corps in Emmaus, Pennsylvania. While Schneck's job requires him to wear a uniform, his personal style is never more than a heartbeat away.

Schneck and a few high-ranking assistants sport *Star Trek* officers' badges on their uniform pockets, just like Dr. McCoy in the original TV series. "I thought that they'd be a neat addition to the uniform," says Schneck, who picked up the $5 pins as gifts for his ranking officers at an Emergency Medical Services convention.

Does the chief worry that the pins detract from his authority? Not at all.

"I'm not really a uniform person at heart. I've always been of the philosophy that if you're a really good leader, you don't have to wear a neon sign that says you're in charge," he says. "Most people respect you for your skill."

---

confined to one genre of clothing doesn't mean that there's no room for being yourself."

Accessorize. While you might not be able to veer far from the suit and tie required at work, you can express the inner you through your accessories—starting with your tie. If you have to wear one, you may as well choose one that reflects your individuality. Accessories are often underrated and even neglected by men. The secret to using them to your advantage is appropriateness.

"You have to be comfortable with how you look and the reaction that you're going to get, but you always need to be appropriate," cautions Marvin Pieland of Saks Fifth Avenue Club for Men. "It's possible to be appropriate, be your own person, and not be a cookie cutter of what everyone else looks like."

Emanating Sex Appeal

How to Be the Featured Attraction

It's nice to have style. Children adore you, men respect you, domestic animals rub against your shins.

There's another side of style, however, that may matter more. It's a side that we're loath to acknowledge, mostly because we're not scoring particularly well in it. It's sex appeal.

"I think when we're young and are becoming sexual beings, we want to be seen as attractive, for our own personal satisfaction and to attract others," says Marvin Pieland of Saks Fifth Avenue Club for Men.

"Once you reach a certain age, especially if you're married, physical attractiveness doesn't seem as important," Pieland adds. "Unless you become divorced. I see that all the time. Then you realize how important looks are once you're back in circulation."

Want a second opinion? Ask the doctor.

"There's no question. Outward appearances are our calling card to the world. They're the first and most accessible part of your image that people see, and people will make judgments about it," says Dr. Ross E. Goldstein of Generation Insights.

Beauty ... Beast?

Remember going out as a teen? You spent a huge amount of time preening before you left home. Why so much emphasis on looking good? Because it mattered. You knew that girls were judging you by your appearance.

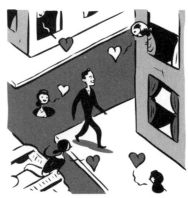

Placing such emphasis on looking good was normal. And natural. And it still is, despite how superficial it may sound. As men, we keep unnaturally quiet about the importance of looking good, because outside adolescence, it's usually viewed as vanity, a character flaw. But that denies the basic nature of life as an animal. "There's no question that attractive behavior is how a successful species adapts. It's evolution, and it's important on a deep biological level," says Hendrie Weisinger, Ph.D., a psychologist, business consultant, and author of *Anger at Work*, *Nobody's Perfect*, and *Dr. Weisinger's Anger Work-Out Book*.

The Science of Sex Appeal

Beauty may be in the eye of the beholder, but according to science, that's more idealism than realism. Science suggests that beauty is really hardwired in our genes and ingrained in our psyches.

"When I started my dissertation work in psychology, people believed that men were above physical beauty," Dr. Goldstein says. "The fact is that attractiveness is one of the most powerful factors in your image."

Reams of studies back this up. One well-known study of college students at the University of New Mexico found that students with the most symmetrical bodies were perceived to be the most attractive. Students whose left and right sides differed by just 1 to 2 percent were found to be more attractive than those who differed between 5 and 7 percent. The prevailing theory is that symmetry implies healthier genes, and our internal mating machine, knowing this, subconsciously drives us in that direction.

In her book *The Complete Idiot's Guide to Dating*, Judy Kurianski, Ph.D., a sex therapist and radio personality from New York City, neatly breaks down the chemical side of attraction.

Among the most common chemicals, or hormones, involved in sex appeal, she says, are adrenaline (the rush), oxytocin (the cuddle chemical), phenylethylamine (natural-high chemicals), and the endorphins (the pleasure chemicals).

Our concept of beauty also is influenced by society. How else can you account for the fact that 42 percent of all *Playboy* Playmates between 1953 and 1996 had blond hair, and almost half had hair that cascaded past their shoulders? Sociological influence works on men, too. Men of power, that is, men who are rich and famous, are generally viewed by society as the most sexy. That's a basic research premise of David M. Buss, Ph.D., psychology professor at the University of Michigan in Ann Arbor and author of the book *The Evolution of Desire*, who surveyed more than 10,000 men and women from 37 cultures on six continents and five islands.

There are psychological factors in sex appeal as well. What rings the "attract-o-meter" for one woman might have everything to do with what's rolling around in her head. She may, for example, feel that a model man is loud, aggressive, and abrasive, because her father was like that. She may be predisposed to the scholarly, sensitive type if her first love was like that and she's subconsciously seeking to find him.

Tools of the Trade

Maybe you don't have much control over whether your eyes are more or less symmetrical, whether you're bringing in six figures a year, or whether the woman that you'd love to love has somebody else in mind. You do, however, have direct control over how appealing others find you. Realize that sex appeal involves connecting with others on an

A Pickup Line by Any Other Name . . .

Forget her sign. Asking is a sign for her to steer clear of you. And forget about the time. If you can't afford a watch, or have nothing important enough to necessitate owning one, she won't give you the time of day anyway.

Herein lies the dilemma. You want to break the ice but don't want to get frosted.

The problem, says Dr. Ross E. Goldstein of Generation Insights, is that in delivering an opening line, you must appear natural in the most artificial setting. You're trying to get someone's attention without drawing too much attention to yourself.

What do you do?

"This isn't going to sound terribly profound, but the truth is that men need to understand the importance of self-disclosure when meeting a woman," says Dr. Goldstein. That doesn't mean telling her about your vasectomy. It means sharing something innocuous about yourself so that you don't appear overly interested in her.

"When you see a woman you want to meet, asking for her name is intrusive. Just giving her your name is not—it's self-disclosing," Dr. Goldstein says. "Most times, that's enough to get her to say her name in return."

instinctual level. Sexy people are magnets, for men and women. "In a sense, you're presenting yourself in a way that pulls me toward you," Dr. Weisinger says. "You're sending out cues, almost like flirting. It's called charisma.

"Sex appeal is bonding. Does the person have a good sense of humor? Is he able to make you laugh? Is he sincere? It's emotional," Dr. Weisinger says. By realizing its importance, you'll be more likely to make the most of your sex appeal.

While physical attraction plays a healthy

role in sex appeal, you're not condemned to solitude if you look more like Chris Farley than Chris O'Donnell.

"All is not lost if you're not attractive," Dr. Goldstein says. "While looks might be important at first, what's behind your looks makes the most enduring and flattering impression." Here's how to be sexier and more desirable.

Humor her. Women find a man with a good sense of humor sexy. And it's not just because he can make her laugh. "Beyond displaying a playful, easygoing attitude, a sense of humor conveys a social presence, which translates into high status," says Dr. Buss. Being funny in front of others shows confidence and an ability to be on top of things without being uptight. But don't run out and buy a joke book. The sexiest way to convey a sense of humor is to learn to laugh at yourself and to find humor in everyday life.

Don't brag. True self-confidence is a turn-on. But there's no surer turnoff than exaggerating your power, sexual adeptness, or athletic prowess. "Women are quite good at distinguishing false bravado from real self-confidence," Dr. Buss says.

Be sensitive, not simpering. It has become a cliché: Women go for the sensitive guy. And there's a certain amount of truth behind the hype. In one study, women looked at a set of responses to questions answered either from a masculine point of view or an "androgynous" viewpoint—meaning a mix of both feminine and masculine traits. The women rated the androgynous male as more favorable in terms of intelligence, morality, dating, and mating potential. But don't don that Ziggy Stardust outfit or try to get in touch with your feminine side just yet. A little bit of vulnerability goes a long way.

"As the feminine side grew, sexual attractiveness declined," says study author

---

Appealing Lingerie

If you want to boost your sex appeal with a special someone close to you, try giving her something close to her: lingerie.

"Women are complex creatures. We're very hard to shop for," declares Joyce Baran, vice-president of merchandising and design for Smoothie, the Strouse, Adler Company in New Haven, Connecticut. "But sexy clothes are the most wonderful gift that you can give. It's the closest thing to her body."

The problem is that many men find shopping for lingerie to be intimidating at best and embarrassing at worst. "Most men in a lingerie shop look mortified or embarrassed beyond belief," says Ellen Jacobson, vice-president of merchandising and design for Goddess Bra Company in Boston. "Clerks are waiting for you. Since you really don't know much about lingerie, they'll take you to the most expensive item and work down from there."

To avoid being taken to the cleaners, here are two things to keep in mind.

Robert Cramer, Ph.D., professor of psychology at California State University in San Bernardino. That's because, for all the talk of making men more sensitive, the truth is that "women admire men who have firm beliefs, take control in financial or career decisions, and protect them when they feel threatened," Dr. Cramer says. The key is to exhibit emotional sensitivity without exhibiting helplessness.

So how do you walk that line?

- Do: Admit when you're wrong or ask for directions when you're lost. Feel free to tear up a little during a Meg Ryan film. Express it when you're feeling hurt or sad. Show some emotional fortitude when bad times hit.
- Don't: Act helpless to get out of doing something that you don't want to do. Get

Remember whom you're buying for. Buy what she'll like, not what you like. Pay particular attention to eye appeal and color, Jacobson says. "What colors does she normally wear? Black is good for most people, but really fair-skinned women should wear blush tones," she says. As for eye appeal, don't rule out anything that isn't fishnet. Women love diversity in their sexy underwear. Silk, satin, even cotton can be sexy.

Size things up. This is one area where size really does matter in the bedroom. Your best advice is to ask her to write down her sizes and keep them in your wallet, says Marie-Helene Miller, designer and chief executive officer of Bamboo Lingerie in New York City. "It's easy to forget because there are so many sizes to keep track of for women," Miller says.

When in doubt, consider a gift certificate or keep your receipt. The second-worst thing to do is to buy the wrong size. Too big, she'll feel skinny, too small, she'll feel fat. What is the worst thing to do? "Buy her a push-up bra. It sends the wrong message," Miller says.

of Love. "And that signifies whether he is willing enough to provide resources for her in the future."

Watch the mirror. A sure sign that your sex appeal is working is if you find yourself and the other person "mirroring" body language. For example, you're speaking with an attractive woman at a bar. Naturally, you lean forward as you speak. If she is doing likewise, you're probably on the right track. (If she is leaning away, you are not making progress. Brush your teeth and try someone new.)

Be an equal-opportunity flirt. Few things perk you up like flirting. As adults, especially married adults, we forget how delicious the fruits of flirtation are. We forget how to verbally fence. To dodge, parry, and be foiled.

"How you flirt is particularly important. Some people, like salesmen, for example, may be natural flirts because of their jobs. They like people, regardless of whether they are attracted to them," explains Princess Jenkins of Majestic Images International.

The secret, she adds, is realizing that "part of flirting is acting." In other words, it's supposed to be embellished and ornamental. Just practice on everyone.

defensive when you're in the wrong. Chicken out after you've made a commitment. Brood, sulk, or play hurt to get what you want.

Be nice to children. This is a surefire way to increase your sex appeal. Displaying affection toward children signals to women that you'll be a great dad. In one study, women were shown slides of one man in three different situations: standing alone, being nice to a baby, and ignoring a distressed infant. Women reported being most attracted to the fatherly type. "Even a woman uninterested in having kids will notice whether a man is caring toward children, because it suggests whether he is a caring person in general," says Helen E. Fisher, Ph.D., an anthropologist at Rutgers University in New Brunswick, New Jersey, and author of *Anatomy*

Act your age. "People yearn for youth," says Brad J. Jacobs, M.D., a plastic and reconstructive surgeon in private practice in New York City.

What this boils down to in sex appeal is this: The better you take care of yourself, the younger you'll look and the more desirable you'll appear. Exercise, eat right, and diligently reduce stress. Pay apt attention to your wardrobe to keep it from dating you. And don't try hard to act younger than you are. Be natural. Wearing a toupee, showing the world your underwear waistband, and saying "dude" won't work for most of us.

Carrying Yourself with Elegance and Grace

The Dynamic Duo of Style

Life on the arid plains of central Niger is harsh, but the nomadic Wodaabe people find time to host tribal beauty contests. Contestants preen for hours in preparation. They dress in tightly wrapped skirts, adorning themselves with elaborate jewelry, headbands, and turbans. They line their eyes with kohl, shave their hairlines, polish their teeth, and color their faces in yellow makeup to accent their noses and eyes. They dance all night to prove their grace and are poked, prodded, eyed, and ogled by friends, family, and judges until a winner is chosen.

Wodaabe beauty contests sound a lot like our own Miss America pageants. Except for one thing.

All the contestants are men.

Polish and Poise

While we don't hold male beauty pageants, those same attributes—elegance, grace, beauty—cherished by the Wodaabe are coveted in our society, too.

But when we talk about elegance and grace, we're talking about something much deeper than looks or image, says G. Bruce Boyer, a private and corporate image consultant in Bethlehem, Pennsylvania, and author of *Elegance* and *Eminently Suitable*.

"Style is an outward assemblage; it reflects lifestyle. Elegance is internal; it's your

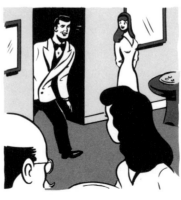

confidence and comfort in yourself, your look, your smile, your demeanor," says Boyer.

Here are some hints to help you convey the essence of elegance and grace, whether you're in box seats at the ballpark or in the box at the opera.

Make an entrance. Whether it's at a cocktail party, a bustling convention center, or a crowded restaurant, the way you move through a room can convey a sense of elegance and grace, even to those who merely see you from afar. "Some people walk into a room. Other people enter it," says Princess Jenkins of Majestic Images International. "Most of us have walked into a room and walked past three people we knew without saying hello because we didn't notice them. That's because we walked into the room, we didn't enter it."

To make a grand entrance, Jenkins suggests the following tips.

- Pause after you walk through the door.
- Survey the room quickly with your eyes, acknowledging whom you know at the far end first.
- As you walk toward them, scan nearby, nodding and acknowledging people close to you, offering warm greetings and engaging in chitchat.
- Continue working the room until you catch up with the people you know at the far end. By then, you will have made a favorable impression on those you chatted with—as well as those who just observed you.

Warm up. Appearing socially warm and approachable instantly boosts your gracefulness quotient. It starts with the basics: smiling, maintaining eye contact, listening attentively, and being sincere.

"It's what your mother taught you. If you're a good conversationalist, have good etiquette, and mind your manners, you're more likable," Jenkins says. One tactic to convey sincerity is to ask people about themselves and ask their opinions. Most people love to talk about themselves and will adore you for asking.

Call on your expertise. Men considered elegant or graceful usually are well-versed on just about any subject. Since we can't be experts all the time, fit in tidbits of your expertise when appropriate. If you know a thing or two about fine wines, share some trivia during cocktail hour. If you're not an expert, become one on a topic that's likely to come up.

"If you go to formal cocktail hours a lot, for example, learn all you can about escargot. Just don't fake anything or seem pretentious—people appreciate knowledgeable people, not phonies or know-it-alls," says Leon Hall of International Apparel Mart and The Fashion Association.

Excel at introductions. You'd be surprised how many people bungle an otherwise easy opportunity to look genteel. Here's a formula to follow for flawless intros.

- Graciously interrupt your current conversation, using the name of the person you're talking to.
- Introduce the newcomer by first and last name. Add some personal details.
- As the newcomer and the person you were talking with shake hands, reciprocate using the same approach.

For example, "Excuse me, Tom, I'd like you to meet Bill Smith. Bill's an attorney at Blindem and Bilkem." [Shake] "Bill, Tom Jones. He's a professor at Whassamatta U."

Be good at chitchat. Small talk is the mainstay of many formal and business-social get-togethers. If you're not good at making small talk, scan the newspaper before you leave home. It'll give you something to lead with.

You Could Have Danced All Night

We asked swing dance teacher Jim Zaccaria, who volunteers with the Philadelphia Swing Dance Society, Dean Constantine, owner of Constantine Dance Studio in Minneapolis, and Gretchen Ward Warren, dance professor at the University of South Florida in Tampa and author of *The Art of Teaching Ballet* and *Classical Ballet Technique*, what dances a man of style should know. Here are the top seven picks.

1. *Country line dancing.* "You don't need a partner, you learn the basics of every type of dancing, and it doesn't have any feminine stereotypes to scare you," Warren says.

2. *Ballroom dancing.* The box step, one-two-three waltz, and fox-trot are dances that you'll do at every formal affair you attend.

3. *Jazz dancing.* À la jazz musicals. Contemporary, athletic, fast-paced, hip.

4. *The hokey-pokey and chicken dance.* Yes, they're cheesy, but you'll see them at every wedding that you'll attend for the rest of your natural born life.

5. *Ethnic dancing.* "Folk dancing, like the polka, is really fun," Warren says. "You'd be surprised how big polka is. There's a vast underground subculture." If that's too scary, learn ethnic and religious dances that are important to you, such as the dance to the Jewish standard Hava Nagila.

6. *Modern fast dancing.* Just because the polka's hard to do to Snoop Doggy Dogg.

7. *The tango.* If one dance alone can stand you out from a crowd, it's this. But it's not for everyone. Very complex. Very difficult. Way cool.

And again, ask questions—people love to talk, and they might feel just as awkward about chitchat as you do.

"Don't try too hard, though, or you could come off as patronizing or insincere. People want sincerity, not schmooze," cautions Dr. Jeff Livingston of Cisco Systems.

Expressing Yourself

Keys to Communication

Remember writing in invisible ink as a kid? You used lemon juice, and after the juice dried, you held your note over a warm light bulb and watched brown, crusty letters appear. Personal style is like that: There's the obvious message, and there's the secret message underneath. Most of us aren't aware of the messages that we're sending, let alone the secret messages.

"Your style is exactly what others say it is, because in the business world and in our personal lives, perception is everything," says Dr. Hendrie Weisinger, a psychologist and business consultant. "Personal style is defined by the observer, and if you're not aware of this, it could be to your detriment."

You could be saying all the right words, but your body language and facial expressions may be sending an entirely different—and even contradictory—message. If your body is saying one thing, and your mouth another, rest assured that people will take the body language as the truth. The goals of stylish communication, then, are to speak with clarity and eloquence and to make sure that the rest of your body is giving the same message as your words.

Riding the Self Express

So you want to communicate with style? Here is some expert advice on the art of verbal communication.

Match words with gestures. Don't let your eyes, arms, shoulders, or feet counter your words. Face your conversation partner squarely; don't let your eyes wander, toes tap, or hands play; and match your expressions and body movements to your words. If you are saying enthusiastic words, for example, your face and hands should be reacting differently than if your conversation is deep and poignant. Most of all, don't let your body say, "I'm not really interested in this conversation." You do that by shuffling, looking around, and fidgeting. If you want out of a conversation, stay focused on it until you can politely excuse yourself.

Hold back to get ahead. One of the keys to expressing yourself effectively is timing, says Michael R. Losey of the Society for Human Resource Management.

"The problem with most people is that they come on too strong in the beginning," Losey says. "They're so intent on expressing themselves that they don't realize that it's not always what you say but when you say it that matters. My advice is to be cordial and polite in conversation or a meeting but to hold back on your important thoughts until the group needs a conclusion or consensus."

Grin and wear it. The easiest way to improve your self-expression is to improve your facial expression: Smile.

"A lot of speakers, for example, concentrate so intently on their speech that they forget to smile or laugh at their own jokes," notes David Wolfe of The Doneger Group. It happens in normal conversation, too, he says.

"It's okay to feel nervous when you're talking to someone or a group of people, but don't let it keep you from appearing warm, friendly, and sincere," Wolfe says. Smiling also:

- Changes breathing patterns, which may oxygenate your brain and improve your mood.
- Makes you sound better. In a study at the City University of New York,

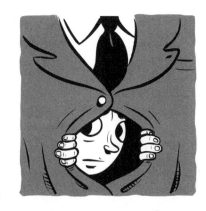

psychologists found that people can tell when others speak with a smile, because they sound happier and more sincere.

- Lends credibility. Another study found that people who doled out punishment were most lenient on smiling people.

Lend an ear. Nature gave you two ears and one mouth so that you can listen twice as much as you speak. Yet, "people often underestimate the importance of being a good listener," Dr. Weisinger says. "Listening attentively and showing empathy—putting yourself in the speaker's shoes—are vital to making a good impression."

While listening may not seem to directly aid in expressing yourself or your views, it does. Attentive listening implies that you're sincere and that you care about what the other person is saying. Listening shows understanding and good manners. "Plus," Dr. Weisinger adds, "it keeps you out of my-way-or-your-way power struggles."

Be a wordsmith. The words you choose to convey your thoughts say a lot about who you are. Whether something's *pernicious* or *stupid* or *deleterious* or *bad* can signal how intelligent you're perceived to be. Pay attention to your vocabulary and choose your words carefully. Collect new words like you'd collect stamps by buying a good vocabulary-building workbook, taking a vocabulary class at a local community college, or by keeping a list in a notebook at home of new words that you've learned. But be careful: Throwing around big words when simple words will do also can send a message, and it's not particularly flattering. You can come across as pretentious, pompous, or worse—especially if you use words when you don't understand their true meaning.

Speak in sentences. If we wrote, you know, on paper—no really, on computers because that's how we write, most of us

---

Accentuate the Positive

You're educated, well-bred, and well-read. But when you open your mouth, you're afraid of sounding like an inarticulate rube.

Having an accent can be a man's greatest handicap in expressing himself—if he lets it. It's true that non-native English speakers and people with geographic dialects—like New Yorkers or Southerners—are subject to occasional prejudice, but speakers with accents are more often victimized by their own self-consciousness.

"The biggest hurdle is in the mind of the person. If a man considers his accent a barrier, then it *is* a barrier," says Louise Elerding of the Association of Image Consultants International and The Color Studio.

"What speakers with accents don't realize is that most people love to hear accents," Elerding says. "We're attracted by something that sounds exotic. We listen more carefully, so the accent becomes an advantage."

---

anyway—as we spoke out loud, like, no one would ever read again because it would drive us, you know, nuts trying to follow the theme, and besides, it would scare us half to death because we'd appear, you know, well, *stupid*. And that's not how we want to come off when we communicate. So if you want to sound intelligent, try to speak as you write. Use clear, short sentences, without all the "ands" and "buts" and "you knows." Let people hear the punctuation—the commas and the periods—because the most listenable speakers are those who speak in grammatically correct sentences.

Let your gaze linger. When talking to a group, talk to individuals. "Pick someone in the first row and focus on them for five seconds," Losey says. "Then do the same for the third row, fifth row, and so on. Now you're talking to people, not a group of heads or the back wall."

Culture and Style

East Side, West Side, All around the Town

Think culture clash, and you think international—the arrogant U.S. businessman in Tokyo, the goofy U.S. tourist in Paris, the boisterous, drunken U.S. party boy in Tijuana.

All those "ugly American" stereotypes may have some basis in truth. But for most of us, they're beside the point—most of us won't be flying to Europe or Japan anytime soon. The problem is ugly Americans in America. As anyone who has traveled the United States can tell you, we're so diverse *within* the United States that culture clash is as likely to occur at home as abroad.

"Look at the guy who comes from Phoenix to a meeting in Manhattan. He's got his string tie on, his light suit, and boots," says Michael R. Losey of the Society for Human Resource Management. "He might be totally at home in Phoenix or Texas, but he'll stand out like a sore thumb in New York City."

Fitting In with Style

A man of style knows how to be comfortable in all cultural situations, be it attending a Bar Mitzvah, eating at a Japanese restaurant, having drinks with a Southern gentleman, or going to a Mexican-style birthday party. This is not easy. It requires not just an open mind but an inquisitiveness about the people and cultures around you. And it requires that you get out of your routine and try new things—be they strange new foods, a different approach to

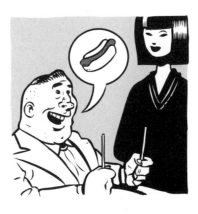

negotiating, or toughest of all, talking less and listening more. Here are some ways to become a universal mixer without compromising your style or individuality.

Play with food. Most cross-cultural events involve eating. You'll make a strong impression—good or bad—with how you handle yourself at the dinner table. Fortunately, this is an area in which you can practice on a regular basis. Most every city has a diversity of ethnic restaurants—use these to learn the foods and eating styles of the cultures that you likely will be encountering in the future. Learn to use chopsticks. Try the various soups and appetizers. Fear no food. Having a well-developed, worldly palate is not only a clear sign of a stylish, confident man but also enormously enjoyable.

Listen carefully, speak frugally. When in a new cultural situation, be a student. Observe how those around you are eating, interacting, and speaking. Don't try to dazzle your hosts with endless monologues; let others do the talking until you have a good understanding of the rules of conversation. Even then, understand that you are an outsider; just because others are being boisterous doesn't mean that you can be loud and lewd, too.

Perceive how you will be perceived. While you might not exactly lose a deal because you talked turkey in your snakeskin boots, know that business acquaintances—and just about everyone else—will be judging you based on your cultural differences.

If you talk with a southern drawl or thick Brooklyn accent, for example, people will judge you on it. What are your best approaches to remedy these prejudices? Don't mask your own cultural traits, but be willing to adapt how you operate to the other party's style. And do whatever you can to make the focus of the interactions the business deal itself, not the presenter.

Walk on the mild side. When it comes to dress, always err on the side of conservative. If you're not sure what to wear for that big talk with the California computer firm, stick to the tried-and-true: dark blue suit, white shirt, conservative tie. Boring? Maybe. Appropriate? Always.

Don't appear superior. Another advantage to dressing conservatively is that you won't condescend. Even accidentally. You never want to be perceived as superior by people you're doing business with, unless, of course, you're being consulted for your superior skills or knowledge. In other words, the $1,000 Brooks Brothers suit that you bought on the Upper East Side of Manhattan may actually alienate you in Topeka, Kansas, says nationally renowned image expert, syndicated columnist, and author John T. Molloy in his best-selling book *John T. Molloy's New Dress for Success.*

Don't be provincial. In cross-cultural encounters, it's small-minded to constantly tell stories about how things are where you live. Stop yourself from comparing food, weather, and the like to your home location. If your New York City hosts take you to a seafood restaurant, for example, don't comment on how the fish compares with that in your home town of San Francisco. Why? Your goal is to fit into the situation; constantly pointing out that you are an outsider defeats you. It also appears small-minded and arrogant.

Be true to yourself. Don't boast about your culture or home region, but don't deny it either. Be true to who you are. If you're from New Mexico, go ahead and wear a turquoise ring. If you are an orthodox Jew, wear your yarmulke proudly. Just don't flaunt your uniqueness—show it naturally, with dignity.

Sometimes, Molloy says, people expect your image to be a certain way, and it behooves you to understand that. For example, say that you're a Wall Street financial wizard called out to the Midwest to talk about the Big Board. Or say that you're a maverick computer guru in Seattle brought to the East Coast for programming. Under these conditions, you'd want to look every bit your role: The financial wizard would reek of Wall Street. The computer geek would reek of latte.

A Foreign Affair

Imagine expanding into a new market and finding that the name of your product translates into "jackass oil."

It happened.

Or imagine selling a car with a name that translates into "small penis." It happened, too, to Ford Motor Company when they attempted to sell the Pinto in Brazil. (They later changed the name to Corcel, Portuguese for "horse.")

Then there's the time shoe manufacturer Thom McAn sparked a riot in Bangladesh. Their nearly imperceptible "Thom McAn" insignia on the sole of their shoes looked so much like "Allah" in Arabic that outraged Muslims thought the shoe company was committing blasphemy. Especially since the foot in Bangladesh is considered particularly unclean.

We'd like to give you 10 steps that'll keep you from making a fool of yourself overseas, but we can't. Nothing personal. It's just that it's impossible to make blanket statements about fitting in in a world as diverse as our own.

Your best advice is to arduously learn what you can about all the countries and cultures with which you'll be doing business. A good book we can suggest is *Kiss, Bow, or Shake Hands* by Terri Morrison, Wayne A. Conaway, and George A. Borden, Ph.D.

Fitness and Style

Shaping Up Your Body and Image

Al works 12 hours a day at a top accounting firm. He brings down a pretty penny and sports $1,000 Armani suits to show for it. Yet his idea of a crunch has more to do with numbers than exercise.

Bruno's a part-time personal trainer and bouncer. He works out two hours a day but can't afford anything that's not off a sales rack at Kmart.

Which guy has maximum style?

Both—and neither.

"It's a strange fact of fashion, but men who spend hours and hours working out don't tend to have jobs that allow them to dress real well, while men who spend all their time making money don't spend enough time in the gym," notes David Wolfe of The Doneger Group. "The irony is that, with the right paycheck, you can buy clothes to disguise your body. Or, if you're in really good shape, even bad clothes look good on you."

But the issue isn't just how well your clothes look on you. A man of maximum style has the stamina to stay at the top of his game throughout the workday. He moves easily and with grace from the tennis court or golf course to the boardroom. And that means that he makes time for fitness in his life.

Exercising Self-Esteem

No one ever said that you had to look like Adonis in

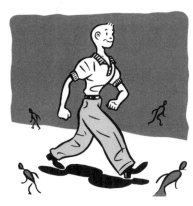

Levi's. Rather, just being in slightly better shape than you are now can add a polished finish to your appearance—and personality, says Dr. Hendrie Weisinger, a psychologist and business consultant.

"An outward appearance of confidence and pizzazz comes from inner feelings of self-esteem," explains Dr. Weisinger. "When you feel good about yourself—about your body, about your health—it shows on the outside. When you look and feel good, you show the world in everything you do."

There's more: Exercise ameliorates attitude. A University of Illinois study of 20 college students—15 of them men—found that 30 minutes of aerobic exercise at 55 to 70 percent effort increased positive feelings and decreased negative feelings of anxiety.

Feeling good and looking good. Sounds like a man of style to us. So if the only exercise that you've been getting is climbing the corporate ladder, try these tips.

Clobber corpulence. Your first step along the exercise-image path starts with fighting fat. Consider that one in three Americans is overweight, and that by the time they reach their sixties, 42 percent of all American men are overweight. While the fat-cat look signified wealth and power in the old days, today it's the opposite: The heavier you are, the less credible you may be perceived to be.

"Weight is one of the criteria that people use in judging your overall professional appearance," says Michael R. Losey of the Society for Human Resource Management.

"Interviewers want to see that your weight is in proportion to your height," Losey says. "Anything more is thought to implicitly signify some type of character flaw."

Live long. Want to be on the cutting edge of fashion several times over? Live long enough and everything you own will be in vogue more than once. Exercise is your ticket to long life, according to a study at the Cooper Institute for Aerobic Research in Dallas. Of 25,341 men studied for more than eight years, those in the worst shape were 1.5 times more likely to die than fit men. Physically active men lived longer even when they had risk factors, such as high blood pressure, high cholesterol, or a bad smoking habit.

Shake things up. Exercise is the fastest way to fry a dead-fish handshake. Do this to be a "handyman."

• Stand upright, with your hands by your sides and your palms inward. Hold a weight plate in each hand by grasping the raised edge of the plate with your four fingers and pressing your thumb against the flat side of the plate. Find a weight that you can handle for 10 repetitions. Straighten your fingers to lower the plate. Now close the fingers raising the plate as high as you can. Do this with enough weight to finish three sets of 8 to 10 lifts.

• Squeeze a tennis ball or rubber handball/racquetball while talking on the phone or stuck in traffic. If you want high-tech, go to a sporting goods store and buy a spring-loaded grip trainer or some silicone rubber, grip-strengthening putty.

Improve your standing. A commanding presence (read: good posture) is one of the first three things that people notice about you. (The other two are hair and eyes.)

"Your standing, your presence, and your posture help make your image," says image consultant Ken Karpinski. Therefore, spending time in the gym working on your upper body reaps big rewards. Pay attention to your back, chest, abdomen, and shoulder muscles: They're

Building Muscle—And Confidence

It's not only common sense that if you look better, you'll feel better about yourself. It's also science.

In one study at the State University of New York College at Brockport, 57 people were divided into two groups: One group lifted weights for 16 weeks, while the other group completed a physical education theory course. Sure enough, it was the weight lifters who boosted their confidence, along with their biceps.

The sports sociologist who led the study, Merrill J. Melnick, Ph.D., explains why the exercise group fared better: "You may see yourself as inferior if you're unhappy with your physical self." By building a little muscle and losing a little fat, he says, you can improve your feelings about your body and yourself.

One reason why weight training may be so effective in bolstering your self-image is that it gets results fast. In addition to being able to see muscle growth and improved muscle tone, you can detect progress easily. "You know in two weeks when you can lift more weights on a machine," says Janet W. Rankin, Ph.D., associate professor in the exercise science program in the Department of Human Nutrition, Foods, and Exercise at Virginia Polytechnic Institute and State University in Blacksburg. That's a little easier to measure than gains in aerobic fitness from exercises such as running or bicycling, she says.

the ones that keep you standing tall. They're also the ones that fill out your suits and define a man's masculinity. Doubt it? Consider one Canadian survey that found that wimpy chest muscles are the second-biggest source of angst in a man's appearance, right after a chubby waistline.

Food and Style

You Are What You Eat

It would be criminal to picture Kojak without his trademark lollipop. Or James Bond, Agent 007, without a martini (shaken, not stirred, of course). And you'd have to be at sea a long time, sailor, to picture Popeye's pal, Wimpy, without a juicy hamburger in his hand (for which he'll gladly pay you Tuesday).

What do these guys have in common? Okay, they aren't real. But the connection that each character made between food and style certainly is.

Style, Well-Done

What you eat or drink says a lot about you. In some cases, like the TV detective Kojak and his ever-present lollipop, it helps define an image.

"It's like that for some of us, too," says Louise Elerding of the Association of Image Consultants International and The Color Studio. "Lots of us know someone who'll only eat strawberry ice cream. Or someone who adores pizza. Or someone who drinks only red wine."

In this sense, food becomes an integral part of the image that others have of you, Elerding says. Through time and repetition, people associate you with what you regularly eat and drink. Think King Henry VIII, think giant drumstick.

Food also augments your image. This happens because certain foods have picked up stylish connotations all their own. Caviar, escargot, and champagne, for example, all smack of affluence, if not opulence. When you associate yourself with these types of foods,

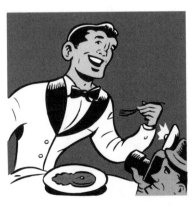

their connotations—both good and bad—will rub off on you.

"You really can be judged by what you're eating and drinking, especially in a major city like New York City, where you're made very aware of trendy food and drink all the time," says Leon Hall of International Apparel Mart and The Fashion Association.

Here's how food and drink can make the most of your style.

Obey your thirst—and hunger. "This is a pet peeve of mine: the man who's so inhibited that he drinks a martini because he's afraid someone's watching," says Elerding. "If you're really in the mood for a beer, order a beer.

"Part of having style means knowing who you are and what you want and not being ashamed of it," Elerding says. "I'm on a quest for honesty: When I'm with a group of professionals, it's refreshing to see someone order the beer that he wants instead of a fancy 'power' drink that he thinks he should have."

If you want a martini, of course, the same applies: Order it, Elerding says, even if the rest of the group is drinking beer.

Drink incognito. That said, you can always take the alternate route and eat or drink to set an image specifically for the occasion. "I used to live in Paris, and I'd give a bartender there about 10 American dollars to keep a martini glass filled with water and an olive for me," Hall says. "I made out well, because I had the look of a martini, without the adverse side effects the next morning. Plus people wondered how I held my liquor so well." So if you're at a cocktail party mingling with the martini crowd but don't like vermouth, pull a Leon Hall: Disguise your beverage. Classy bogus beverages include water and an olive in a martini glass, orange juice in a tumbler instead of a screwdriver, no-alcohol beer in a chilled beer mug, Coca-Cola on the rocks instead of a rum and Coke. You get the idea.

Eat for the health of it.

"Healthy eating is in," Hall says. "I eat very little fat and hardly any cholesterol. It's not only good for you but also very much in vogue."

According to a survey by Food Marketing Institute in Washington, D.C., and *Prevention* magazine, more than 50 percent of food shoppers have made major dietary changes for health reasons in the past three years, and 58 percent say that they almost always read nutrition labels before buying. A healthy diet gets no more than 30 percent of its calories from fat, though some experts advocate 20 percent or less. Ten percent of your calories should come from protein and 60 percent from carbohydrates. On average, most men ages 20 to 60 get 34 percent of their calories from fat, 47 percent from carbohydrates, and 15 percent from protein. (The remaining 4 percent comes from alcohol.)

What does eating healthy fare say about you? It shows that you're knowledgeable about nutrition and that you care about your health and appearance. Those are stylish traits in anyone's book.

Fear no food. Ethnic foods tend to be healthiest, especially Greek, Italian, and Asian eats. Moreover, knowing something about ethnic cuisine makes you look refined—something that never hurts your image, says Caitlin Storhaug of the National Restaurant Association.

"Imagine how you'll look if you take an important client or date to an Ethiopian restaurant not knowing that you'll have to eat without utensils," Storhaug says. Just being able to navigate a foreign menu or skillfully manipulate chopsticks when you must lends an air of culinary credibility.

Take out an insurance policy. If you're not sure what to expect at a particular restaurant, ethnic or no, call ahead and ask questions. If it's Japanese, for example, ask if chopsticks are mandatory. Ask if there's private

Ignorance Is Never in Style

You'd think that they'd know better, but it just isn't so. People with various diseases know little more about diet and nutrition than you do—even though this information directly affects their well-being.

Researchers at Ohio State University studied more than 2,700 Americans and found that people with cancer, osteoporosis, high blood pressure, and heart disease had eating habits just as poor as everybody else. "We found that just having a disease was not a strong motivating factor to adopt good dietary practices," says Denis M. Medeiros, Ph.D., professor of human nutrition and food management at Ohio State University in Columbus and the study's lead author.

The only people who seemed to take a stronger interest in their diets were those who had high blood cholesterol or diabetes.

seating. Ask what the wine list is like. Ask if you'll have to eat with your hands or wear a stupid-looking lobster bib. Knowing what to expect up front saves face and makes you look decisive when the waiter walks up.

Enjoy food with flair. Some ethnic foods boast distinctive flair and appeal. They're fun, classy, and worthy of exploration, Storhaug says. Her picks include Japanese steak houses and sushi bars, and Ethiopian, Indian, and Thai restaurants.

"These places are great because they place so much emphasis on presentation. People want entertainment, atmosphere, and good presentation with their food. Stuff that you don't get at home," Storhaug says.

"Oh, and if you want to look good on an important date," she adds, "here's something that you must know: Nothing will get women talking about a date in the worst way as taking her to someplace that only serves octopus."

Aging in Style

Be a True Prime-Time Player

As a young man, you were so sure of everything. Who you were. What you wanted. And how you were going to get it. Then, one day, you gazed in the mirror and saw a middle-age guy who looked surprisingly like your dad, and you wondered what happened. This time of deep questioning, of reassessment, that usually occurs between ages 38 and 43 can be wrenching, leaving in its wake disillusionment and broken relationships. That's the pattern commonly referred to as midlife crisis or middle-age crazy. Many of us have known guys who fell into the trap, trading in their wives for younger women and their old family station wagons for newer, sportier models. Heck, some of us have *been* that guy.

Realizing that the days remaining in our lives grow ever fewer than the days that have passed can be unsettling. But the key to aging with style and grace is to accept and embrace who you have become. Instead of a time of emotional upheaval, this necessary midcourse adjustment can be a joyous time of self-discovery and inner peace. And a man who has a firm grasp on who he is and is at peace with himself is going to be a man of great style, a man admired and respected by other men—and women.

The Distinguished Gentleman

If you want to live long and well, you must embrace life. That is the conclusion of Ben Douglas, Ph.D., professor of anatomy at the University of Mississippi Medical Center in Jackson and author of *AgeLess: Living Younger Longer.* Dr.

Douglas has studied scores of centenarians and found that attitude is the single most important factor in reaching that coveted milestone.

"Regardless of race, religion, socioeconomic background, even their diets, in my research the people who age the best all seem to share similar characteristics," Dr. Douglas says. "They all have a good sense of humor; they don't take life too seriously. They tend to be active, having worked hard every day of their lives. And they also tend to be forward-looking people. Rather than looking back at what they have done or didn't do, they focus on what's ahead, whether it's the election or a baseball game or seeing their grandchildren."

Here are some things to keep in mind as you look ahead.

Conquer the world. Look at life as a never-ending, always-unfolding adventure. In action, this means always reading new books, trying new restaurants, traveling to new places, taking on new sports or hobbies, even changing jobs every now and then. Just always keep moving forward. For there is nothing more appealing or commendable about a mature man than his having a sense of fun and adventure.

Be a mentor. As you look around the office, you notice how young the other guys suddenly seem. You have two choices: Resent them, and spend your time bitterly grousing about how much better the office used to be before it was overrun by these damn kids and their computer games. Or embark on a journey of mutual learning. Become a mentor, sharing with the younger men your knowledge and experience—things that they could never get from any computer program or book. And open yourself to what they can teach you about the new technology that's revolutionizing the workplace.

Enjoy fatherhood. Maybe one of the reasons that you look like your dad is that

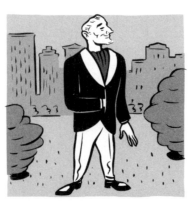

you're now a dad yourself. Again, attitude is everything. You can sit around reminiscing about how much fun you used to have when you were young and free, or you can throw yourself into fatherhood with the same spirit and verve that you once reserved for Saturday nights. Be a part of your kids' lives, especially their play. Take them to the park. The zoo. The museum. The ballpark. Show them—don't just tell them—that learning is fun and that new experiences are exciting.

Look Sharp

Sure, your youthful looks may be a thing of the past. Your hair may be gray or gone. But the question isn't what you've lost. It's what you've found—the character, wisdom, and experience that only living can bring.

"The issue is not how you can look like 30 forever," says Princess Jenkins of Majestic Images International. "It's really how you can look yourself but still look current and not dated, regardless of your age."

Here are two suggestions.

Throw a fit. It's important to go through your wardrobe periodically in order to make sure that all your clothes still fit.

"You'd be surprised how many men hold on to the same suit for years because they think that it fits," Jenkins says. Retire your duds when buttons strain, you can't move your shoulders easily, your pleats or suit vents bulge, lapels and collars bow, you need to hold your breath, your long sleeves look short, or people ask, "Where's the flood?" when they see your high-rise pant cuffs.

Play the classics. Some guys seem older because the style of their clothes dates them. What was stylish for one year in the early 1980s, for example, might look absurd on you today. To avoid such a mistake, stick with

---

Riding High

Much like carbon-dating, counting tree rings, or taking core samples of Earth sediment, estimating the age of a man lends itself to a similar, albeit less scientific, method: how high on his hips his waistband falls. "I've wondered about that, too," laughs Jerome E. Oppenberg of Wardrobe Wagon. "It seems that the older a man gets, the higher his pants get."

Although unsure why, Oppenberg speculates that it's because most men sport such big stomachs when they age—their waistbands have to move above or below it. "Maybe it's more reassuring with your pants over your paunch," he says, "or else you feel like they're falling off."

Author David Feldman tackles this oddity of age and style in his book *Why Do Clocks Run Clockwise? and Other Imponderables.* After talking with the American Apparel Manufacturers Association, Feldman concluded that the most logical explanation is that pants were cut higher before the 1960s. Therefore, most men 50 and above never wore pants that were designed to ride on the hips. The pants they grew up with were "high cuts" designed to ride on the waist. Hence, older men are probably uncomfortable starting to wear their pants lower at a ripe old age.

---

classic, enduring clothing styles: solid-colored or pinstripe suits; pullover, cotton-knit, polo, short-sleeve shirts; oxford-style, button-up, long-sleeve shirts; solid-colored dress slacks (with or without pleats); casual khaki chinos; and high-quality sweaters and turtlenecks.

"I have a double-breasted blue blazer, and every time it wears out, I buy the same exact thing—you can't go wrong," says Jerome E. Oppenberg, president of Wardrobe Wagon in West Orange, New Jersey, a special-needs clothing store for the elderly.

Putting It All Together

Measuring Success on Your Own Terms

Next time you're at a computer, crunching numbers in Excel or checking out the latest pictures on the Elle MacPherson Web site, consider exactly what it is that you're looking at. Because what you see is not what you get.

A picture on a computer screen is actually thousands of tiny dots called pixels lumped together so closely and so precisely that they create a distinct image. The naked eye sees people, symbols, words, and icons. Or, if you're lucky, an equally naked MacPherson. But under a magnifying glass, all you see are thousands of very tiny colored dots.

Your image is exactly like this. Although seemingly whole on the surface, it's actually the aggregate of many disparate components, the pixels. You've already arranged the pixels of your image without even knowing it. The question isn't whether you have style. You do. The question is whether you have your maximum style. The only way you will is by taking apart your image and examining it pixel by pixel.

"You might not be able to manipulate the broad brush strokes, but you can exert reasonable control over the details," says Dr. Ross E. Goldstein of Generation Insights.

A Matter of Appearances

Here's a secret, one that you should have been told

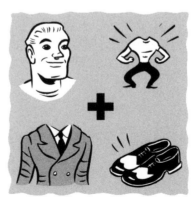

when you were a kid. Heck, it's one that *we* should have been told when we were kids: Looks count, appearances matter. And while you know that you shouldn't judge a book by its cover, everyone thinks that he can. And does.

"I was in a store once, and my six-year-old said that the clerk looked like Brad Pitt. The clerk said that he wished that the girls thought so, but he did look like Pitt," says sociologist Dr. Jan Yager.

"Because the clerk didn't think that he looked like Pitt, it was a great example of the power of self-perception versus public perception," Dr. Yager says. "Because of the difference between self-perception and public perception, there are people in this world who get passed over because they have substance but no glitz. It's a shame."

Scientific studies and style experts support the conclusion that appearances make a difference. Here are some examples.

• A study of 2,500 male and female lawyers by the University of Texas at Austin found that attractive attorneys earn as much as 14 percent more than their less handsome peers.

• A study of college students at the University of New Mexico found that students with the most symmetrical bodies were perceived to be the most attractive. (Researchers also found that female students having sex with more symmetrically built men were more likely to climax. Oh, to be young and symmetrical!)

• Nationally renowned image expert John T. Molloy describes in his book *John T. Molloy's New Dress for Success* an early study that he conducted regarding raincoats. Molloy asked 1,362 people to rate the prestige of "twin brothers" who were wearing beige or black raincoats. The brothers were really the same man dressed identically, except for the raincoat. More than 87 percent ranked the man in the beige coat as more successful, because, Molloy concluded, beige raincoats signify upper middle-class. Black raincoats signify lower middle-class.

So maybe we do initially judge books by their covers, and people by the way they dress. Good looks and stylish dress may open doors for men, but what they do once they're inside is up to them, says Dr. Jeff Livingston of Cisco Systems.

"The good news is that most people eventually want to see what's really underneath. Ultimately, they want to know what you're all about," Dr. Livingston says.

The Successful Man

What are you all about? What is it that you want to be known for? The answers to those questions will determine how you judge whether you're truly successful. It's a much tougher standard than clawing your way to the corner office with the windows, or earning enough to buy that Mercedes-Benz.

"Today's man is saying that he will be the judge of his own success—not someone else," says Dr. Goldstein in an attitudinal style study that he compiled for Levi Strauss and Company.

"Today's man is reserving the right to measure success on his own personal terms and less on society's," Dr. Goldstein says. What this means, according to Dr. Goldstein's findings, is that "success is now defined from the inside out. It's how a man feels, not what he owns."

A Cybermodel of Efficiency

Imagine walking into a fine haberdashery and trying on 32 outfits without loosening your belt or unbuttoning your shirt.

Impossible?

Not necessarily. Thanks to computer technology, fashion experts are doing pretty much the same thing now. Fashion designers are literally strolling cyberspace catwalks in ersatz fashion shows to see how their clothes wear and look before the clothes are even made.

According to a June 1996 issue of *New Scientist* magazine, designers at the University of Bradford in England have designed a machine called the Marilyn Monroe Meter that allows them to see how experimental apparel will fare before it ever hits the sewing room. The program replicates on-screen exactly how clothing will look and act on a live model, based on algorithms that account for every flounce, kink, or snag in the garment's design and the qualities of its fabric. The cybermodel flaunting the electronic clothing owes her lifelike behavior to real-life models, whose movements were laser-scanned and also set to algorithms.

What does that mean for you? Well, according to our humble imaginations, it's not too far-fetched to envision a spin-off of this program that allows you to scan in an image of yourself in order to see how you'll look in certain outfits before you even buy them in a virtual try-before-you-buy scheme. The photo-scanning technology is already available, as anyone who reads *Weekly World News* knows. (You didn't *really* think that Elvis was lunching with aliens, did you?) And it would be a great way for men to make one of their most abhorred chores—shopping—a little more hassle-free.

According to Dr. Goldstein's study:

- 71 percent of men say they are fairly to extremely successful.
- 93 percent feel very optimistic about their own futures.
- 45 percent of men like their changing role in society, 36 percent are neutral, and 19 percent don't like it.

Based on Dr. Goldstein's study, the following five criteria are ranked most important in determining a successful man's style.

1. Being a good father
2. Having good relationships with his wife or significant other
3. Being healthy and fit
4. Being socially responsible
5. Achieving balance between work, family, and social life

Judging from the results, "excess, narcissism, and irresponsibility are out. Relationships, healthy living, and balance are in," Dr. Goldstein says.

"The old adage that 'clothing makes the man' is still true. However, dressing for success in today's changing world requires personal style and individuality," he says.

Rebuilding with Style

Here's how to deconstruct and reconstruct the pixels of your personal image.

Take a real interest in people. Looking good is only a part of style. The essence of substance is how you act. That means conducting yourself in a way that would make Mom proud.

"I've saved one advertisement from the early 1960s that shows a guy in a double-breasted blue suit talking to a lady in a babushka with a cleaning rag," says image consultant Ken Karpinski. "Underneath the picture it says, 'You've got style when you know the cleaning lady by her first name.' "

Build from within. Ric Flair, the profes-sional wrestler, epitomizes style in a strangely ironic way: He's a bastion of civility in a sport that thrives on melodramatic machismo and comic-book violence. Throughout his decades-long career, Flair has maintained an image of elegance, even opulence. When he's not in the ring, he's often seen near it surrounded by beautiful women, while wearing a tuxedo and sipping champagne. But despite the Dom Perignon, diamond Rolex watches, sequined robes, and pinkie rings, real style starts on the inside, Flair says.

"It's all a frame of mind. Being built bigger or smaller, being richer or poorer, doesn't have much to do with it," he says. "You can tell that someone has style when they exude inner confidence. You can tell they know that they're doing the best they can in everything they do."

At six feet one inch, 240 pounds, will you argue with that?

Take small steps. We all cut corners in at least one area of our image. Maybe it's rushing through ironing. Or keeping our favorite clothes so long that they don't fit anymore. Maybe you've never learned to dance or never taught yourself how to stop sounding so nasal on your answering machine. Solution? Fix them—one at a time, Karpinski says.

"Putting together, or revamping, your image takes time. It's a growing process, but it starts with the small steps," he says.

Talk it up. Bring up style with people in the industry whenever possible. Root out opportunities to pick their brains. Try to mingle with image consultants at your next chamber of commerce mixer. Frequent fine retail shops and politely interrogate the staff.

"Listen to people who know what they're talking about," says Daniel C. DeCosta, vice-president of North American Operations for Joop! Jeans in New York City. "Especially go to the fine specialty stores. These people are traveling Europe and the world to find out what's cool, what's hip, what's hot, and what's not."

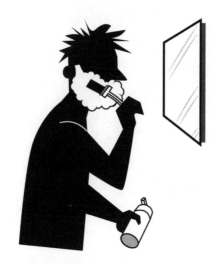

Part Two

Grooming

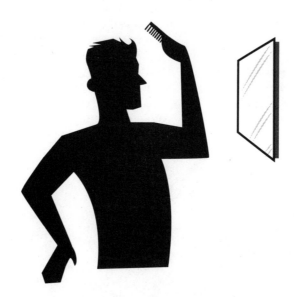

Hair

A Heady Subject

Life is symmetrical. We come in bald. We go out bald. In between is a life of trimming, primming, pruning, and shampooing; of do-ing, dyeing, and blow-drying; of brushing up, down, sideways, and 'round; of training, coaxing, cajoling, and sometimes outright punishing our hair to do as we want.

And why? Because those thin strands—amalgams of keratin (protein) and melanin (a pigment)—say so much about us. Since the beginning of time, hair has been an indicator of a person's position and inclinations. Do-gooder Diogenes, back in ancient Greece, searching for an honest man, made long hair and beard a prerequisite. Ever since the Romans cut the locks of captured barbarians for the slave markets, short hair has been a sign of servitude. Monks and Marines cut their hair to demonstrate their conformity and discipline. On the other hand, long hair has often been associated with free-thinking individualists (a polite way of saying hippie, isn't it?).

"The way we know that hair is so important to men is by how much trauma it causes them when they lose it," says Marietta Baba, Ph.D., chair of the anthropology department at Wayne State University in Detroit.

The Art and Science of Hair Shine

Put a hair under a microscope and it will look like snakeskin—bands of overlapping scales. Hair looks its best when the scales that surround the hair shaft lie flat against it. Then the hair reflects light evenly instead of diffusing it at each scale. Hair shines even more when lots of healthy hairs lie together smoothly, reflecting light off one another. Helping to keep each hair smooth, soft, and shiny is a small amount of oil secreted by a gland attached to each hair follicle.

The key to healthy, handsome hair is to maximize hair shine by managing these two things: the amount of oil in your hair and the quality of those scales. Both face a myriad of challenges, however. Dry air, heat, sun, pollution, chlorine, poorly or excessively used hair products, and even bad brushing technique all ruffle those scales, clog the oil glands, or cause an overflow of oil production.

The retail establishment has responded to these hair challenges with shampoos, conditioners, thickeners, gels, and mousses that smooth scales and increase shine by coating the hair shafts with glossing agents or infusing them with protein. Then, when we use this stuff too much, we buy special "clarifying" shampoos to wash all the accumulation away. It's a big business, this hair thing.

But don't be deceived. In truth, hair care is easy and needn't be expensive. Here are the essential hair-management tasks.

Wash often. Shampoo daily unless your scalp is exceptionally dry. In this case, rinse with water one day and shampoo the next. Men tend to overuse dandruff shampoos, leaving hair overly dry. Use dandruff shampoo when a problem emerges, then switch back to a gentler shampoo when the problem dissipates. Even if you don't have dandruff, switch back and forth between a couple of shampoos every few weeks to avoid buildup.

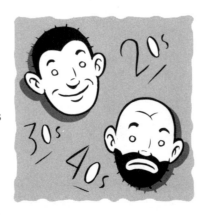

Condition it. A good-quality conditioner will thicken and smooth your hair, giving it shine and bounce and character. After shampooing, rub conditioner in and leave it on for a minute before rinsing.

Dry carefully. Towel it down first, then blow-dry using medium to high heat but low speed or airflow. Don't overdry; stop while the top layer is still slightly damp.

Consider doing a dab. It is not unmanly to put a little mousse or gel in your hair to help keep it in place. The trick is to get the right product for you. Some gels are impossible to detect; some make your hair seem permanently wet; some give just a slight bit of support; others plaster your hair to your head. Obviously, pick the one that gives you the look that you like. Each product has different ways to apply, so read the instructions. But typically, when your hair is still slightly wet, you'll put a teaspoon or so of the glop in one hand, rub your two hands together to spread it out evenly, then rub it into your hair, concentrating on the front and sides, which are the most likely to lose their shape as the day progresses.

Comb gently. Use your fingers, a hair pick, or a wide-tooth styling brush to desnarl after shampooing. A bristle brush dragged through tangled hair can cause lasting damage; only use bristles when you are brushing your hair into place.

Match your hairstyle to your face. There's a science to hairstyles. Much of it hinges around the shape of your face. For example, if you have a big nose, don't part your hair down the middle—it's like having an arrow pointing at your schnozz. Also, if you have a square face, let your hair grow a little longer in the back to give the illusion of a longer face.

The truth is that there is little way for regular guys like us to know all these tricks. See a good hair specialist. Have him recommend a style based on your facial structure, the quality of your hair, and the image that you wish to project. Leave professional jobs to the professionals. (And smartest of all, pick one trustworthy professional and stay with this person. Every six weeks is a good timetable to keep for haircuts.)

The Seasons of Your Hair

Hairstyles change. Lengths go up and down. Popular cuts have about as long a life span as a political campaign promise. But there are some generalizations that we can make. Here's what you can expect from your manly mane through the ages and stages of your life.

The Thick Twenties

These are the salad days of your hair. It's young and healthy, so it can take the abuse that you dish out. And you *do* dish: the long hours of beach volleyball—without head covering, using whatever shampoo you find in whatever shower you find yourself in the next morning, letting it grow too long for its own good. But even in these halcyon hair days, there is this foreshadowing of things to come: Between the ages of 18 and 29, some 15 to 30 percent of men experience some degree of hair loss, according to the Chicago-based American Hair Loss Council, a nonprofit organization. Treat healthy hair well in its heyday and you may have it around to enjoy later on. Use gentler cleaners low in astringent detergents but high in emollients, says Matt Teri, director of product development worldwide for all Aramis products, based in New York City.

The Transitional Thirties

Your career is moving into the fast lane. Your relationships are going through re-evaluation. Your hair seems to have a head of its own. And don't look now, but your hairs are thinning—all of them. That is, each separate little sucker looks like it has lost weight. This means that your hair dries faster, is less shiny, looks flatter, and feels less inviting to fingers of the opposite sex. Because the thinning happens on top of your head, one solution is to let it grow out on top but keep it trimmed at the back and sides. Meanwhile, from ages 30 to 39, as much as 40 percent of men experience hair loss. So if you're going to try any of the chemicals that claim to fight balding—like minoxidil (Rogaine)—this is the time because the chances of success are better for guys who've been balding less than five years. But don't get your hopes up, advises Coleman Jacobson, M.D., director of dermatology at the Baylor Hair

Research and Treatment Center in Dallas. "Minoxidil and other surface treatments don't seem to be panning out well. Though it's been very profitable for such makers as the Upjohn Company, I'd call it hope in a bottle."

The Fading Forties

Your professional goals are in sight. Your home life is relatively settled. But things on top are a little unsettling. It's time to face the bald fact: 45 percent of men ages 40 to 49 experience hair loss. The shower drain is looking hairier than your pate. Despite the disappointment of Rogaine, you still have options for maintaining a semblance of your former bushy-haired self. First and foremost is working with what's left by re-evaluating your haircut. The last thing you want to try is "the toilet seat top"—combing a few lonely strands across the barren frontier of your forehead—so called because you (or the wind) can lift it like a toilet seat. "This style draws attention to the problem rather than covering it up," says Rick Brockhoff, head of the barber department at the College of Hair Design in Lincoln, Nebraska.

Instead, go short, not long, says Teri. "Keeping it shorter will give the appearance of thickness and fullness," he says. "If you layer it, there are more ends of the hair showing. There's more surface area for the light to reflect off of. Long hair looks flatter, you see more space between the strands, and you can see the scalp more easily."

The Resigned Fifties

At work, your 20 years of labor are bearing fruits. At home, an end to mortgage payments is within sight. On top, what's left (by this age, 55 percent of men will experience hair loss) is turning gray, the result of the early retirement of our follicles from producing pigment. Some men mind this, but most men don't. If it bothers you, hey, if Dennis Rodman can dye it, so can you. "The basic chemistry of hair coloring has not changed much in the last 50 years," says John Corbett, Ph.D., vice-president

of scientific and technical affairs for Clairol in Stamford, Connecticut. "Hair is tough stuff, an extremely strong fiber that can withstand the effects of dyeing without suffering any noticeable structural damage." He offers these tips.

Go pro. A professional colorist is going to do a better job than you will at home. It may cost you in the hundreds of dollars and several sessions, but chances are better that in the end you will turn people's heads—for the right reason, not the wrong one.

Go toward the light. If you're "dyeing" to do it yourself, the main mistake that amateurs make is that they dye their hair too dark. Try it in shades. Use a shade a little lighter than the color that you want your hair to be. "It's easier to make it darker than lighter," Dr. Corbett notes. First-time users don't take into account the shade of their own hair. He recommends starting with the lightest shade and working your way up.

Pick your speed. If you dye at home, there are three choices. Gradual hair coloring, like Grecian Formula 16, works over several weeks. This gives you a chance to regulate the shades over time. It also means that the guys at work won't notice so quickly. The second is demipermanent—for instance, Men's Choice. It could last from three to six weeks before you need a refill. If you don't like what you look like, you can go back to gray. The third is permanent—an example is Just for Men—and has more peroxide than the other product. This one's for keeps.

The Satisfied Sixties

The command generation: You're in charge at work and at home, and as far as your hair goes, with 65 percent of you experiencing hair loss, you've generally learned to let go— though you may be willing to hold off the inevitable one more time with hair replacement surgery. If so, here are some guidelines from Sheldon Kabaker, M.D., associate clinical professor at the University of California, San Francisco, Division of Facial Plastic Surgery.

Monitor costs. There's some misleading information out there because of the competitiveness of the market. "To have enough work done to make a difference, hair replacement surgery could cost between $8,000 and $20,000 after all is done," says Dr. Kabaker. Comparing this lifetime investment to the cost of a new car might put this expenditure in perspective.

Monitor risk. If the judgment of the surgeon is wrong, the hair could fall out. There are cases of detrimental side effects—visible scarring among them—but Dr. Kabaker puts the risk of hair restoration no higher than dental restoration, which is not very high. As a safeguard, check the surgeon's reputation and longevity of work within the area that he works. Be wary of transient surgeons or clinic chains that don't check out.

Keep expectations realistic. Though a hair transplant is "good for 90 percent of balding men," says Dr. Kabaker, it may not be advisable for the remaining 10 percent. "A medical physician would turn down someone who has unrealistic expectations," says Dr. Kabaker, like wanting a full shock of natural-looking hair. Men who have been balding since their twenties or men whose balding pattern has left them with an inch-wide horseshoe-shaped border of hair might not be good candidates.

Okay, so hair replacement surgery is not on your must-do-in-this-lifetime list. There's always the toupee. Just don't call it that. "The word has negative connotations," says Anthony Santangelo, president of the American Hair Loss Council.

Call it what you will—hairpiece, hair unit, hair system, or hair replacement—but Santangelo estimates that as many as seven million American men wear some sort of non-

surgical hair replacement.

The fibers for most hairpieces are made of a modified acrylic by a company in Japan. They are fire-resistant, keep their curl, and won't fade—which is more than you can say for

Off the Shelf

Ten million hair products, just one head. Here's what you need to know about all those hair products that you see on the drugstore shelves.

Clarifying shampoo: Used to clean away buildup from other hair products.

Conditioner: Treatment applied to wet hair after shampooing, then rinsed out. Adds vitamins, moisturizer, shiner, protein, detangler, and more to your hair.

Gel: Glop that holds hair in place. Good for styling short hair. Put on wet hair, it dries hard, leaving a wet look. Put on dry hair, it takes off the fluff and is less noticeable.

Glosser, shiner, polisher, laminator, glass: A potion filled with silicone or oil that you rub onto your hair to smooth it and make it gleam. Just a few drops will do you; more than that and you'll look like an oil slick.

Moisturizing products: Term for shampoos, conditioners, and treatments that soften dry, brittle hair. Many contain glycerin, which helps hair grab and retain moisture.

Mousse: A foaming conditioner that helps hold hair in place. Better for wavy, longer hair.

Spritz, spray gel: A lighter, liquefied gel, sprayed onto hair as a mist. Keeps it in place. Good for all hair textures; can be applied to wet or dry hair.

Thickeners, volumizers, body builders: Ingredients found in shampoos and conditioners; also stand-alone products that infuse hair with proteins or coat hair with polymers or waxes to make it seem thicker.

pieces made of human hair, says John R. Moot, president of National Fiber Technologies Limited in Lawrence, Massachusetts, one of the few hairpiece manufacturers based in the United States. You'll pay from $500 to $2,000—though a hunk of that piece of change will pay for the national advertising that you see on TV and in newspapers, he adds.

The most important thing is the fit. You can tell that it's a bad fit when you can tell that it's a hairpiece. "If they fit well, you can't tell that they're wigs, and you'd be surprised at how many men walking around are wearing them."

Hairpieces attach to a man's scalp in one or a combination of ways: two-sided tape, clipped to the existing hair, or "permanently" attached to the back of your natural hair (although as your hair grows, the attachment loosens).

But the real trick to wearing a hair piece is in your head, not on it, says Moot: "You have to be relaxed about it. People who know you will know that it's not all yours."

Finally, once you have surrendered to hair's evolutionary process, you may want to take complete command by shaving it all off. At least you'd be in impressive company: R.E.M. lead singer Michael Stipe, George Foreman, Willard Scott, and Michael Jordan are just a few of the approximately 35 million men in the United States who are bald or balding.

"Bald is a sense of pride," says John T. Capps III, a printer and founder of Bald-Headed Men of America, a support group based in Morehead City, North Carolina, which has amassed a membership of 20,000 since its founding in 1973. "It's a badge of distinction. It takes a real man to be able to take some ribbing and then dish it right back." The organization's motto is "Bald is beautiful."

And that's not all that it is. "Half the

Dandruff: The Yeast You Can Do

Everyone has a little dandruff. Your scalp dries, you itch, small bits of dead skin fall off. Not pretty, but no big deal. Many of us have a slightly bigger problem—dandruff caused by a yeast called *Pityrosporon ovale*. In 20 percent of the population it leads to dandruff, also known as seborrheic dermatitis. If you suffer from dandruff, it's some relief to know that you're not alone. "People are itching to see me," half jokes Dr. Coleman Jacobson of the Baylor Hair Research and Treatment Center.

The basic remedy for recurring dandruff, says Dr. Jacobson, is fairly simple: Use an antidandruff shampoo that suppresses that yeast. The active ingredient you're looking for is selenium sulfide, as in Selsun Blue. Follow the instructions on the label. Give it two to three weeks. Here are some other options.

Try rotating shampoos. Sometimes your hair and scalp build up a kind of immunity to the same shampoo used daily. Rotate several dandruff shampoos for better results.

women we talked to said that totally bald is really a turn-on," says Dr. Baba. "It's like the guy is saying, 'I'm so confident in my sexuality that I don't need any hair.' " So much for Samson. Plus, adds Dr. Baba, why tiptoe around it: A bald head is a pretty graphic phallic symbol.

Odds and Split Ends

Finally, here are some expert tips to help you get through even the baddest hair day.

Play the part. Wondering which side to part your hair on? Ask a friend to check your crown. If the crown is on the left, then you should part your hair on the left. Or just comb your hair straight back; it will fall naturally to the side you should part it on. Part the wrong side and your hair will lump and wave where it

Trim out stress. Several conditions that commonly cause dandruff are all influenced or aggravated by stress. Just knowing that dandruff may be related to stressful situations in your life may reduce worrying about what's causing the dandruff and eventually reduce the flaky problem.

Shed sunlight on the matter. Some sunlight may temper the growth of the yeast, according to Jerome Shupack, M.D., professor of clinical dermatology at New York University Medical Center in New York City.

Extend an olive branch. Dr. Shupack recommends this home remedy: Massage a few drops of olive oil into your scalp after shampooing at night, cover your head with a shower cap, and shampoo again in the morning.

Live better through chemistry. Nonprescription hydrocortisone lotion can relieve the inflammation that leads to dandruff. A stronger prescription cream version is also available. For stubborn cases, resort to ketoconazole (Nizoral), a prescription antifungal shampoo.

have hair that's just as proudly distinctive as they are. They should care for their hair heritage as much as their other traditions.

• Asian men generally have thick, coarse hair that should be cut and thinned out every month or so to keep it looking good and healthy, suggests Brockhoff. "A cheap cut will show on this type of hair," he adds. "Conditioning is also important, since it's dry hair."

• African-Americans face other problems, depending on whether their hair is curly or kinky, says John Atchison, owner of John Atchison Hair Salon in New York City. For one thing, because of the curl pattern, natural oils secreted by the hair have trouble sliding out along the shaft to the ends. That also detracts from the hair's natural sheen. So it's important to shampoo with a conditioner that will keep the hair well-oiled. Atchison recommends shampooing at least every other day. He also suggests getting hair cut by sectioning it with scissors and comb rather than a clipper so that the ends can be cut. Otherwise your hair will look dull and frizzy. As for the various methods of manipulating those kinky curls—texturizing, relaxing, loosening, straightening—just remember to replace the protein that these chemical treatments rob from the hair by using various conditioners and oils.

• Latino men should keep their hair longer, suggests Angel Martinez, a stylist at Francis Hair Salon in Union City, New Jersey, who also styles hair for on-camera talent at Univision, the Secaucus-based Spanish TV network. "Because our hair is so straight, there's nothing that you can do with it when it's short," he says. "It sticks up like a porcupine—not attractive." Keep it at least three inches long. Also, he adds, some Latino men are adding highlight to their hair to lighten the color. "It softens the features of our faces," he says.

shouldn't. "Parts make for a more groomed, more conservative look," says Gillian Shaw, senior barber at Vidal Sassoon Salon in New York City. "It makes hair look flatter." She suggests that men with curly hair forgo the part. Just use your fingers to fluff it into place after you shower and let it dry naturally.

Slim up with sideburns. If you want to create the illusion of a longer, thinner face, bring back the burns, says Brockhoff. Not the big Elvis-style handlebars—even they couldn't hide his pudginess in his later years—but the more discreet version, ending parallel with the bottom of your earlobe. Curly-haired men should avoid sideburns, adds Brockhoff: "They get out of control."

Honor your roots. Men of color—whether of Asian, African, or Latin descent—

Glasses and Contacts

Looking Good While Seeing Well

The days are long gone when men who wore glasses also had to wear monikers like "bookworm" and "four eyes."

"Men in glasses can be very sexy," says Margaret Dowaliby, O.D. (doctor of optometry), professor of optometry at Southern California College of Optometry in Fullerton and author of 10 books on optics, frames, and lenses.

"Glasses frames are just as much a part of how a man expresses his style as anything else he wears," adds Dr. Dowaliby. "You should even consider different frames for different outfits and occasions."

Here's Looking at You

Before they are fashion accessories, first and foremost eyeglasses are corrective devices for people who would walk into walls if they didn't wear them.

To be precise, "glasses" is a misnomer. While about 12 percent of corrective lenses are still made of glass hardened by heat or chemicals to meet U.S. Food and Drug Administration standards for impact resistance, the rest now come in a variety of other materials. Plastic lenses made of a hard resin command 71 percent of the market. They are lighter and more impact-resistant than glass, but they're thicker and scratch more easily. Polycarbonate lenses, which make up 17 percent of the market, are light and thin, made of the same plastic used for bulletproof windows.

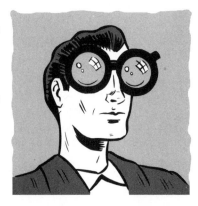

"This is the finest plastic that you can buy," Dr. Dowaliby says. Though four to five times as impact-resistant as other lenses, they scratch easily. Aspheric lenses are lightweight and thin; they minimize magnification so that your eyes don't look like a frog's behind the lenses. High-index lenses are the newest kind, recommended for strong prescriptions; they're lighter in weight and thinner at the edges.

There also are specialty lenses. Photochromic lenses grow lighter and darker according to available light. They can screen out up to 85 percent of light at their darkest and 10 to 15 percent at their lightest. Polarizing lenses reduce or eliminate glare from roads, water, and sand.

Surface coatings can make plastic and polycarbonate lenses scratch-resistant. An antireflection coating applied to both glass and plastic lenses reduces glare for dusk or night driving and strong indoor artificial lighting—great for those of us who deal with the flashing lights of those annoying paparazzi. Ultraviolet (UV) coatings block hazardous UV radiation from the sun.

If you wear prescription glasses, chances are that they're single-vision lenses, which help you see all distances. As you age, you may need bifocal lenses—which contain two prescriptions. One corrects for nearsightedness (you can see near but not far), the other for farsightedness (the opposite). If you don't want the world to know exactly how bad your eyesight is getting, progressive addition lenses make a gradual invisible transition from one power lens to the next, obliterating that telltale line between the bifocal lenses. On the other hand, you can go for the mature look and wear Ben Franklin–style half-lenses, as does *60 Minutes* reporter Ed Bradley.

If you would rather not deal with glasses at all, and wouldn't mind changing the shade of your baby blues—or greens or browns, as the case may be—soft contact lenses come in two kinds of tints that can cosmetically change the color of your iris, says Charlotte Tlachac, O.D., associate professor of optometry at the University of California at Berkeley and chairwoman of the contact lens section of the American Optometric Association. A light tint can significantly change the shade of blue and green eyes, while making brown eyes darker. Opaque tints consist of a series of dots that make brown eyes darker but will make "light eyes look grotesque," Dr. Tlachac says. They are not recommended for people with larger-than-average pupils. Tinted lenses will increase the cost of soft lenses by about 40 percent, says Dr. Tlachac; opaque lenses will double the cost.

The Frame-Up

Seeing well is one thing. Looking good is another. "People need to understand that the frame that they choose makes a statement about them," says Clifford W. Brooks, O.D., associate professor of optometry at Indiana University in Bloomington and author of *System for Ophthalmic Dispensing*. If you want to be on top of the latest frame trends, look toward Europe, says Dr. Brooks. "Whatever is going on there will be in vogue in the United States five to six years later," he predicts.

You can use frame shapes to repeat or counterbalance your facial lines and shapes, suggests Dr. Brooks. "Ideally, you want balance," he notes. So the hard edges of a square face can be softened by round glasses. A roundish face will look good with squared-off frames. Men with a heart-shaped face should wear frames with heavy temple pieces that draw attention away from their pointed

Made in the Shades

Sunglasses sales rose from 160 million pairs in the United States in 1985 to 276 million in 1995 (of which 45 percent were male buyers)—a 73 percent jump in a 10-year period.

"It's no secret that many men like the masking characteristic of sunglasses," says Jim Pritts, president of the Sunglass Association of America and vice-president of development for Revo Sunglasses in Sunnyvale, California. "Men particularly like them because they can gawk at women without being caught."

If you're one of the few who actually buys them more for the functional benefits of blocking harmful ultraviolet (UV) sun rays than the fashion statement they make, you may be in for a surprise, says Calvin Roberts, M.D., an ophthalmologist at the New York Hospital–Cornell Medical Center in New York City. He asserts that there is no way for consumers to be sure that they are getting UV protection—even if sunglasses are labeled "UV-absorbing" or "UV-blocking."

"There is no government regulating power for the classification of sunglasses," says Dr. Roberts, so there's no way to be sure that sunglasses that you buy on the street, for example, have UV protection. He suggests buying only from reputable companies or from a physician's recommendations.

chins. A man whose eyes are set close together should choose a frame with a clear bridge but a distinctive temple piece to draw the observer's eye outward. A wide-eyed guy needs the opposite, a frame with a low-set dark thick bridge to fill in the space between his eyes. Men with oval faces have lucked out: Almost any style of frame will complement their bone structure.

Beards and Mustaches

Taking It on the Chin

We'll start with the bare beard facts:

- A man's beard grows an average of 15/1,000 inch a day (that's about 5½ inches a year).
- A man's beard contains between 7,000 and 15,000 hairs (the same number of hairs as a woman's legs and underarms combined).
- In an average lifetime, a man will remove 27½ feet of whiskers from his face.
- Some 90 million American men shave an average of 5.3 times a week.
- The majority of men begin shaving between the ages of 15 and 16.

Not only does a beard say it all—masculinity, paternal authority, spiritual leadership, artistic revolutionary, social anarchist, ivy-tower intellectual, and the passage of time (don't forget Father Time)—but also short of dyeing your hair purple, it is one of the fastest ways to change your appearance.

"Beards are an easy way to signal that a man is ready for a change," says Bonnie Jacobson, Ph.D., director of the New York Institute for Psychological Change, adjunct professor of psychology at New York University (both in New York City), and author of *If Only You Would Listen.* "Beards can be a statement of independence, of maturing and risk taking.

"But a beard can play many roles," she adds. "It can make a man less easily seen— you have to knock before he'll let you in. Or it can be the

opposite—a very public signal that you are not one of the crowd."

You have to wonder which of the above motivated one Paul Miller of Rancho Cucamonga, California, to grow a nine-foot mustache, earning him a place in the *1996 Guinness Book of World Records* for having the country's longest upper lip hair. Actually, he told a reporter, what motivated him was none of the above.

Said Miller: "I have fun with it."

Whiskers A-Go-Go: How to Get a Close Shave

The fun part is growing it and playing with it. Shaving it is largely a chore. But a profitable one—profitable, that is, for U.S. razor makers, which shave an estimated $1.2 billion from men for the pleasure of being clean-shaven.

Of all the male rituals, this has to be the most bizarre. We have marveled at the act ever since we could stand on the toilet top and watch Dad masterfully carve up his face. Nearly every morning the majority of our gender genuflect in front of a mirror, wielding a sharp object toward our throats. If you started at the age of 18 and spent 10 minutes a day at it, by age 60 you'd have put in no fewer that 2,555 hours shaving.

When you're ready to take it off—*take it all off*—follow these tips for some smooth shaving.

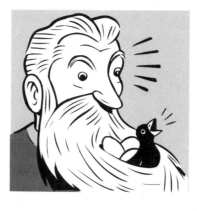

Shave early. Shave first thing in the morning, when your skin is less sensitive, suggests Daniel Rouah, who owns a salon in London.

Wet the whiskers. Gillette researchers estimate that a beard is 70 percent easier to cut after being soaked for two minutes in warm water. That's all the convincing that we need. Water at, say, 125°F will cause the facial hair to expand and soften. Mild soap will wash natural oils and other debris hugging those prickly hairs from the surface of your face.

Lather up. It *is* possible to shave with warm water, soap, a sharp razor, and a rock-solid hand. But why? The water absorbed by the hair quickly evaporates. Lather or gel are like a warm blanket holding in the heat and moisture. They also contain lubricants that reduce friction between blade and skin. For the smoothest shave possible, leave the lather on for two to three minutes before starting, suggests Seth L. Matarasso, M.D., assistant clinical professor of dermatology at the University of California at San Francisco.

Go lightly and slowly. Use a light touch when shaving. This is not a contest to see how close a shave you can get. Or how fast you can finish. We're talking about a sharp object against one of the most sensitive areas of your body—even women's legs and underarms have fewer nerve endings than the face does. "Getting the closest shave known to mankind is going to traumatize your skin," notes Dr. Matarasso.

Shave with the grain. Stroke in the same direction that the hairs grow. Sure, you can shave against the grain and get a closer shave. But two things: (1) So what? It's only going to grow back tomorrow; and (2) Shaving up pushes the hair up. "You're basically training it to grow back down into the skin," says Dr. Matarasso. And that's how you cause ingrown hair and razor bumps.

To look sharp, use a sharp razor. Everyone agrees to only use a supersharp razor, but not everyone agrees on how long a blade remains

Slow: Razor Bumps Ahead

They are the bane of shaving, especially for men of African-American descent. While an estimated 30 to 40 percent of African-American men are plagued by this condition, anyone who has tight curly hair has dealt with razor bumps. The medical term is *pseudofolliculitis barbae.* Most of us call it, simply, ouch!

They are caused when the hair on your face curls and grows back into your skin. Your body doesn't recognize these errant hairs and attacks them as it would any alien, causing inflammation and infection. When you shave over that hair, you're only exacerbating already irritated skin, often causing a break in the surface.

Men who have this condition should start with a clean, sterilized razor, recommends John Atchison of John Atchison Hair Salon, where many of the clients are African-Americans. Here are other suggestions.

- Shave in one direction.
- Don't pull your skin taut to get a closer shave.
- Use a sharp razor with double-edged blades.
- Use tweezers to untangle ingrown hairs, then cut them with your razor or clippers.

Try an aftershave cream that straightens facial hairs. One is Nel's Smoother Skin, an over-the-counter medicated cream that attacks the bacteria that cause razor bumps.

Another topical treatment product, called Tend Skin, was developed by Florida dentist Steven Rosen, D.D.S., who discovered aspirin's potential for drawing buried hairs from the skin so that they're more easily shaved off. He admits he doesn't know exactly how his mixture of acetylsalicylate (the active ingredient of aspirin) and other ingredients works—but it does.

sharp. Rouah suggests that if you use it more than four times, "you might as well break a bottle and use that to scratch your face." Gillette has found that men tossed the company's most durable blade, the Sensor Excel, after 11 shaves. Gillette's disposable razor gets an average of 8 uses. It comes down to a private matter among you, your face, your beard, and your razors. If you tend to draw blood, you've drawn the line on that blade.

Cheek it out. Your cheeks can handle the abuse first. Let the vulnerable areas—chin, lip area, and that most sensitive region of your neck and Adam's apple—soak up as much water and lather as possible before shaving there.

Keep the machine clean. Cleanliness is essential, says Rouah. Rinse the blade with warm water several times as you're shaving.

Beware aftershave. After shaving, one of the worst things that you can do to irritate your just-skinned skin is to slap on some alcohol-based aftershave lotion, says Dr. Matarasso. "They're a no-no," he says. Warm or cold water is fine.

If you insist on splashing on some aftershave, Stephen Schleicher, M.D., director of the Dermatology Center in Philadelphia, says that you should be aware of which kind works best with your skin condition. He offers the following quick guide.

Oily skin: This type of skin can handle the alcohol in aftershaves. It can even benefit from its astringent nature.

Dry skin: Look for low alcohol content and such additives as vitamin E, which moisturizes your skin and helps heal cuts. Also look for another moisturizer containing allantoin.

Acne: Use lotions that won't clog pores (pharmacists know it as noncomedogenic).

Face the Facts

Want to dress up your face the only way you can? Grow a beard or a mustache. You will immediately become part of a male tradition that harks back to the very earliest of times—certainly before Gillette ever hit the scene.

Not only are you making a statement either of independence from all other men or, ironically, of membership in a men-only club but also you are making a fashion statement that can affect the shape of your face.

Covering the bottom half of your face focuses attention on the top half. Specifically, it adds drama to your eyes. A wide and short beard makes a thin long face look stronger. For weak chins, try the Abraham Lincoln look—a thin jawline beard. Find the face shape most like yours in the following list and on your next long weekend or vacation, chuck the blade. Give your skin a vacation, too, and let your manly side come forth.

- Narrow face: full beard and mustache, or hold the mustache
- Round face: lean beard and mustache (connected), keeping cheeks shaved down; beard and mustache (unconnected); or goatee and mustache
- Square face: goatee and mustache; or lean beard, no mustache
- Oval face: standard beard (slightly trimmed along the cheeks) and connecting mustache

Some contain chamomile.

Sensitive skin: Alcohol-free balms with moisturizers such as aloe vera are what you need. Read the small print for licorice root, an anti-inflammatory for razor burns.

Normal skin: Regular guys should still be concerned about removing dead skin cells. Aftershave with alpha hydroxy acids will do the trick. Any of the above can't hurt either.

Colognes and Aftershaves

The Scent of a Man

Think of the rush that your body gets when you smell coffee. A freshly mowed lawn. That's how powerful scent is. Not only do we identify the aroma but also it evokes a memory: mornings in a New York City deli, your father's backyard on a Saturday morning.

To the woman in your life, your scent is just as evocative. Blindfolded, she would recognize your shirts from a pile of unwashed clothes.

"We talk about love at first sight, but we should really talk about love at first sniff," says Alan Hirsch, M.D., a neurologist and psychiatrist with the Smell and Taste Treatment and Research Foundation in Chicago. "Odors from both the environment and other people cause us to have an emotional reaction, and then we make a cognitive decision to rationalize our feelings."

In other words, continues Dr. Hirsch, we assume that people who smell good are good and that people who smell bad are bad. Therefore, you might figure, if you smell sexy, you are sexy. But before you douse yourself with Paco Rabanne cologne, consider this: Men and women perceive odors differently, and what smells like sex to you will most likely not smell like sex to the woman in your life.

And be aware that there is absolutely nothing that says that you have to wear aftershave or cologne to be a man of style. It's entirely your choice.

"Scents for men are getting lighter and more unisex every day," says Michael Skidmore, vice-president of couture clothing and sportswear for Barney's New York in New York City. "But there's nothing wrong with not wearing any. I prefer not to, and I don't feel any pressure to wear one. It doesn't feel natural to me." Skidmore says that the scent of Juicy Fruit gum seems to have become his signature scent by default and that no one has complained yet.

The Science of Scents

Shop for a scent and there are three traditional choices: cologne, eau de cologne, and aftershave. They are differentiated primarily by the amount of essential oil in the mix. Cologne is stronger than eau de cologne (*eau* translates to "water" in French), and both have more scent than aftershave, which is mixed with alcohol. A woman's perfume is the purest product because it has the greatest percentage of scent.

The high alcohol content of aftershave gives it quite a sting. The purpose of that sting is antiseptic; the alcohol cleans and protects the freshly scraped skin. The alcohol also can dry out the skin. Is this a problem for you? Then use a scented facial moisturizer rather than an aftershave, especially if nicks and cuts and acne aren't an issue for you.

These days men's fragrances come in a full range of products, such as deodorants, moisturizers, and soaps. These scents are more

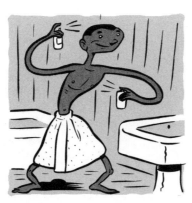

subtle than cologne. How you apply the scent also affects its strength. Splash-ons have more scent than spray-ons, which diffuse the fragrance. If you want to turn one into the other, ask the salesperson for a spray-top that will fit onto your fragrance bottle. They usually have them.

Here are some tips to help you choose and wear the right scent correctly.

Ask for help. When it

comes to picking the right scent, you can't trust your own nose. Instead, trust the reactions of others . . . especially women. "Women have a better sense of smell than men, and younger people have a better sense of smell than older," says Dr. Hirsch. "I always advise men to let a young woman buy their cologne. Or at least advise you on your choice."

Go easy. Once your companion helps you pick the right scent, enlist her advice on how much to put on. "While humans can easily detect a smell for a few seconds, it then becomes invisible to us," says Natalie Hinden-Kuhles, vice-president of fragrance development and evaluation for Revlon. "You want your fragrance to be wonderful and diffusive, not to invade the space of others. Only someone very close to you should notice your smell. It shouldn't hang in the air around you." In other words, if everyone in the office knows that you wear cologne, use a little less.

There is, however, one person whom you shouldn't consult on these matters, advises Chris Tsefalas, owner of Perfume House in Portland, Oregon: the saleswoman in the cologne department. "She's trying to sell you something, not be commended for her honesty," points out Tsefalas. Instead, spray a small amount of the fragrance on your wrist and walk away from the counter. Then, in a few minutes, ask your companion what she thinks of the scent. Or ask for a sample of the fragrance to take home with you and try it over the course of a full day.

Why the wait? Classic colognes have different "layers" of scent, explains Annette Green, president of The Fragrance Foundation in New York City. The first whiff is the top note, which will only linger for a few minutes. It will fade to the heart or middle note, eventually mixing with your own aroma and sweat to create its base. This will last, Green says, for about four hours, depending on how oily or dry your skin is. (Oily skin holds scents longer.)

Come clean. Cologne will not mask the odor of a man who hasn't showered in a day or two. Nor will it cover up the smell of cigarettes. "A man's cologne should smell fresh and clean," Tsefalas says. "In this way he doesn't have to worry about offending people with his odor." But, he adds, you will only smell fresh and clean with cologne if you smell fresh and clean before you put it on. Tsefalas recommends using a glycerin soap, such as Neutrogena, because it won't leave a scent that conflicts with your fragrance.

While slapping on some aftershave is bracing at best, stinging at worst, Green says that it gets men into the bad habit of putting fragrance on a place (your face) that has sensitive skin. Instead, aim for pulse points such as the chest, wrist, elbows, knees, or neck.

Know where you're going. "Men should wear one cologne for day and another, more exotic one for evening," says Tsefalas.

However, Green suggests that you pick a cologne not for day or night but for the occasion. A cologne that smells like citrus or the outdoors is for events that aren't romantic or dress-up, she explains.

There are some places, however, where cologne is not to be worn, and number one on the list is the gym. The scent will mix with your sweat and the odor can become stronger and even downright offensive.

Order room service. She's coming over for the first time? In his research, Dr. Hirsch found that aromas other than perfume often turn people on. "Food scents consistently provide people with a positive memory," Dr. Hirsch says. "Some natural scents, such as lavender and rosemary, have also been shown to relax people." So if she's on her way to your place, don't neglect the way the room smells. Chances are that scented candles or a natural room freshener that reminds her of the sunny days of childhood will make more of a positive impact than cologne.

Buy the best. "You do get what you pay for when it comes to cologne," Tsefalas says. Fragrances contain either real essential oils (from flowers) or chemical imitations of them.

"Before they learn about fragrance, men will pay extra money for a new cologne that gets a lot of press, but eventually, knowledgeable men will choose to purchase a quality product that's well-made," he says. Instead of looking for the cologne with the most hype, suggests Tsefalas, find one that suits the person that you are. Have it be your signature scent, because, as we said before, it's something that the woman in your life will identify with you and you don't want to smell like every other Joe out there.

Keep it cool. If you do opt to spend the big bucks on a fragrance, then make sure that you take care of your new prized possession. To remain fresh, cologne should be kept in a cool, dry place. In fact, don't rule out the refrigerator as a place of storage, says Green.

Fragrance with pheromones. One of the discoverers of pheromones in humans, that magical stuff scientists believe attracts one person to another, is Winnifred Cutler, Ph.D., founder of the Athena Institute in Chester Springs, Pennsylvania. Dr. Cutler has created a product to be mixed in fragrances that is meant to attract women to you, although the women won't be conscious of what's affecting them.

"Fragrance is actually just a carrier of these hormones," explains Dr. Cutler. "You can put Athena Pheromone 10X, my pheromone product, in your aftershave or cologne, and you will experience increased romantic attention and affection behavior." All men and women secrete these hormones, but each person does so in different levels.

"That's why some people just seem to have a certain something that makes them

Alleviating Allergies

There are two ways to be allergic to scent. Your skin can react to the application of fragrance, or your nose can react to the aroma of someone else's perfume.

"Because fragrance formulations are secrets of the industry, we don't know exactly what's in each product," says Mary Lupo, M.D., associate clinical faculty member at Tulane Medical School in New Orleans. "But similar ingredients are found in aftershaves, colognes, and detergents." Fragrances are a leading cause of contact dermatitis, which is characterized by an itchy, red, bumpy rash.

Your dermatologist can give you a patch test for an allergy to fragrances, but if you notice a rash with red bumps or scales or if you itch where you put the cologne or aftershave, then chances are that you have an allergy. "Try putting the cologne on your hands, putting your hands in your hair, and then washing your hands," advises Dr. Lupo.

If you find yourself sneezing when you sniff her hair, or feel your throat closing when her wrist reaches in front of your nose, this, too, can mean an allergic reaction to fragrance. In this case, the only thing to do is kindly ask the woman of your dreams to refrain from using all products that aren't marked "fragrance-free." And remind her that it's her pheromones, not her perfume, that keep you coming back for more.

attractive," Dr. Cutler says.

If you feel that you need a little boost, you might consider using a pheromone-based product. These include Realm for Men, which has a natural pheromone, and Jovan Andron for Men, which contains a synthetic pheromone, according to Green.

Mouth

Flash Your Million-Dollar Smile

She's standing across the room; your eyes meet. What's the next move? It's obvious: a smile. Outgoing, warm, friendly—your mouth will say it all. But if you're afraid to let go with a grin because your teeth are crooked or yellow, well, then . . . there she goes, looking away.

"In many ways your mouth reflects who you are," says Esther Rubin, D.D.S., who has a private dental practice in New York City. "If your teeth aren't clean, then people will wonder about your other hygiene habits. And why don't you bother to take care of your mouth? Do you have low self-esteem? People evaluate you on your looks, and your smile is an important factor in that."

Back to Basics

The keys to a healthy mouth and teeth are brushing and flossing. So here's a pop quiz. It's a variation of the standardized *Gilligan's Island* test used by the finest universities and hospitals. You're stranded on an island. (Whether it's with Ginger or Mary Ann is your call.) But you only have room in your pocket for one item: a toothbrush or toothpaste. Which will it be?

If you chose the toothpaste—for that clean, minty freshness you've heard so much about—you can kiss your chances of getting up close and personal with your fantasy girl good-bye. Plaque is the villain that covers your pearly whites, making them look yellow or brown. "It's not toothpaste that gets rid of plaque, but your toothbrush," Dr. Rubin says. "Toothpaste can help you feel refreshed, but it's not imperative."

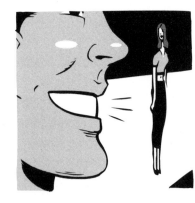

Of course, the bonus is that aside from looking good, if you brush right, you'll also keep your teeth and gums healthy.

"Good brushing technique doesn't just clean the teeth, but it massages the gums," Dr. Rubin says. "Start on the gums, moving in the direction of your tooth, either up or down from your gums. And don't forget to brush your tongue and the inside arch of your teeth."

Dr. Rubin says your best brush bet is a soft, nylon-tipped model with a small head, which will help you reach out-of-the-way spots. "A rough brush can aggravate your gums and cause localized trauma," Dr. Rubin says. In this case, harder is definitely not better.

While mouthwash is a good adjunct to brushing and flossing, says Dr. Rubin, you can live without it. "It helps remove stray bacteria on the tongue and the sides of the mouth," she says. "It's not really cleaning your teeth, but if it gives you a good feeling and lets you feel more relaxed about smiling, then by all means, rinse."

Flossing, for many of us, ranks right up there with eating our vegetables. We know we should do it. But we don't. So here are three reasons why you might want to start. One, you had a poppy seed bagel last week and there's still a black spot stuck between two teeth. Two, that same poppy seed has begun to sprout bacteria. Three, that bacteria is starting to bore a cavity into your tooth. And let's face it—silver looks a lot better in your pocket than in your mouth. The only way to remove that sneaky little sucker is by flossing. "Just do it," says Dr. Rubin. "It should be a habit. It not only removes food but it also removes bacteria that collects daily." And it's the bacteria that causes cavities and gum disease.

Dr. Rubin adds just one caveat: "Do it right." And what is the right way? Start with the floss up into the gum and scrape down each side of the tooth, using a sawing motion as you go along. "You're not cleaning the space between the teeth," Dr. Rubin adds. "You're wiping down the side of the tooth and getting into the gum where the bacteria collects."

Banishing Bad Breath

"It's not as bad as everyone thinks," says Jon L. Richter, D.M.D., Ph.D., a periodontist who opened the first bad breath center in the United States. The Richter Center, in Philadelphia, has served more than 10,000 customers, and Dr. Richter says that most people who have bad breath can easily fix it. And a lot of people who have bad breath don't have it nearly as bad as they think.

"The way to tell if you have a problem with bad breath is if someone tells you or if you ask a friend," Dr. Richter advises. Your own sense of smell can't detect your own bad breath, he says, because it's adaptive, meaning we don't notice an odor just seconds after we smell it. And, unfortunately, there is no self-test for bad breath. "It won't help to breathe into your cupped palms or lick the back of your hand," he continues. "Your breath can take on an odor simply by mixing with air."

The cause of bad breath? "Bacteria that resides on the back of your tongue gets gassy and emits an odor," Dr. Richter explains. The solution? "Clean up the bacteria."

"Think of the bacteria on your teeth. It has to be scraped away, and the same is true for the bacteria on your tongue," Dr. Richter says. "But since a toothbrush can't get all the way back to where the tongue is coated, you can try a teaspoon or buy a tongue scraper."

So why head to a specialist? "I apply a chemical bacteria-killer and scrape your tongue more thoroughly than you can, making the area inhospitable to the bacteria," Dr. Richter says. In fact, controlling bad breath usually requires only a few visits and some homework, not a

lifetime of treatments.

And you can go back to eating garlic, too. While certain foods—especially garlic, onions, alcohol, and coffee—contain chemicals that enter your bloodstream, mix with oxygen, and create a kind of sulfur, for the most part, the odors go away once the food is out of your system. No food will cause chronic bad breath.

So how about all those gums, mints, mouthwashes, and pseudo-medical products that are supposed to keep us clean and fresh? "Well, bad breath does not originate in the stomach as some advertisements say," Dr. Richter explains, "and anything that smells minty is just using one odor to mask another." Products that create a tingly feeling? Those could make the problem worse by drying out the mouth, which leads to the growth of more bacteria, Dr. Richter adds.

Hit the Bleach

Not everyone is born with pearly white teeth. And even those who are will notice that they lose their luster over the years, because teeth naturally darken with age. Like most of the changes that occur as we get older, you can gracefully accept it and concentrate on keeping your mouth clean and healthy. But if it bothers you, there is an option: bleaching.

Although not everyone can be helped by bleaching, "almost everyone will see some sort of improvement in the color of their teeth," says Dr. Esther Rubin, who has a private dental practice in New York City.

Just don't be fooled by the claims of whitening toothpastes you find in the grocery store or drugstore. "Over-the-counter bleaching is bogus," Dr. Rubin says. "Instead, have your dentist customize a mouthpiece and give you a bleaching system to use at home." You'll wear the mouthpiece every night for a few weeks, and the effects should last from one to four years.

Deodorants and Antiperspirants

Taking Control of Sweat

You probably put on deodorant to keep women from smelling you. But over the years numerous studies have found that women are biologically attracted to the natural scent of men, and for good reason. In a small study conducted in Switzerland, researchers found that women were attracted to male body odor that differed from their own. This unconscious awareness of body odor helped them find a mate with a complementary immune system, thus allowing them to create a biologically superior child. Likewise, Dr. Winnifred Cutler of the Athena Institute has found that men's odors have a positive effect on women's menstrual cycles, fertility levels, and menopause symptoms.

"It is true that you shouldn't sweat about whether a woman likes you," says Dr. Alan Hirsch of the Smell and Taste Treatment and Research Foundation. "Her nose will tell her even if she doesn't know why."

But don't think that tossing the Right Guard into the trash will help you land Kathy Ireland. Body odor is a by-product of sweat, and what causes you to sweat largely determines whether you stink.

"Humans sweat through eccrine glands when exercising and apocrine glands when they are embarrassed or sexually excited. Apocrine glands release high-density steroids that have an unpleasant odor. That's why we have a fresh kind of sweat and a smelly kind of sweat," Dr. Hirsch explains.

Apocrine glands are concentrated around your underarms, navel, anus, and pubic area, while eccrine glands—a key component in your body's temperature control system—are embedded in every inch of your skin. Built-up bacteria, which feed on the apocrine gland secretions, are another leading cause of foul body odor (sometimes called B.O.).

Sweat-Fighting Secrets

For both kinds of sweat, the cosmetics industry offers two primary products: deodorants and antiperspirants.

Deodorants cover up bad smells. They rely on chemicals that fight bacteria-caused odor. They also usually have a masking scent, which covers up the smell of your sweat, although you can buy fragrance-free deodorants.

Antiperspirants, on the other hand, work by blocking the sweat from emerging from the pores. If you're a guy who stains the underarms of his shirt, these might be for you. The main ingredients in all antiperspirants are salts, aluminum, or chloride.

Different situations may dictate different choices for you. If you know that you're going to be dripping with sweat because of a workout, then you might want to use an antiperspirant. But if you have a stressful day ahead of you that promises to tax your apocrine glands, you might need a deodorant. Want to play it safe? Use a combination deodorant/antiperspirant. There are plenty on the market.

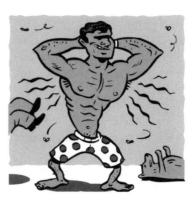

One other note: Spending more money on a deodorant doesn't buy you more protection. The main difference between expensive designer deodorants and those you find on the shelf at your neighborhood drugstore comes down to dollars and scents. If you want your deodorant to match your cologne, then a designer scent might be for you. But realize that the basic chemicals fighting wetness and odor are essentially the same.

Here are some fresh tips to help you K.O. the B.O.

Act quickly. If you do smell your own B.O.—and the odor is unpleasant—repair the damage immediately because "we get desensitized to any odor quickly," says Natalie Hinden-Kuhles of Revlon, makers of Mitchum antiperspirant. "You won't smell it after a while, but everyone else will." Remember that neither cologne nor deodorant will mask a smell that's already there, so if you sniff it, wash it, and then apply something to fight future odor.

Scrub up. Deodorants won't stand a chance if they're being applied to unclean skin. Sure, you wash, but are you using a soap that will fight odor? Antibacterial soaps and deodorant soaps will get rid of the germs that feed on sweat to create smell. "Don't give the sweat something to grab onto," Dr. Hirsch says. "If you clean the area well, then the bacteria's intensity will decrease."

Clean your clothes. You scrub under your arms, put on the deodorant, but then you toss on a T-shirt that still smells, faintly, of body odor. Fabric holds on to odor, so if you notice your clothes come out of the dryer still smelling like a combination of all your scents, find a different detergent. And consider washing your clothes with a detergent that is unscented or fragrance-free. That will cut down on the cornucopia of aromas emanating from you and your clothes.

Cut out smelly food. If your food smells strong, chances are you may, too. Take garlic, for example. Sure it's going to boost your immune system, but it may also be the reason

The Power of the Crystal

Your intentions are good. You throw powder where you should, spray on deodorant where you should, and even though you end up smelling clean and fresh, your skin turns red and uncomfortable. Some skin just doesn't take well to fragrances or preservatives, both of which are found in most deodorants and antiperspirants.

If this is you, then buy hypoallergenic or fragrance-free products, says Dr. Mary Lupo of Tulane Medical School. "This usually means that the fragrance and the preservative have been removed."

The problem, Dr. Lupo continues, is that many consumers think a deodorant or antiperspirant labeled "unscented" is also safe. "Unscented simply means that it doesn't have an aroma that will conflict with your cologne, but it still has fragrance in it to mask the odor of the ingredients."

Some people with allergies use a "crystal," which is a clump of aluminum chloride that acts as an antiperspirant, but not a deodorant. "This is simply the main ingredient of most antiperspirants, without all of the added fragrances and preservatives," explains Dr. Lupo.

But some people are allergic to the actual salt itself, whether it's in a crystal or an antiperspirant. If that seems to be your problem, says Dr. Lupo, try baking powder or baking soda, which can absorb the perspiration, but not deter it.

you smell the next day. Any aroma that overpowers your kitchen will find its way out of your skin, too. Other foods that often contribute to B.O. include fish, cumin, and curry. If you're having an odor problem, try cutting strong spices out of your diet for a few days to see if the smell eases up.

Unwanted Body Hair

Finding Fur in All the Wrong Places

You can be wearing a $2,000 Armani silk suit and a pair of $200 Italian loafers. But if you have protruding nose hair, you might as well be wearing a Wal-Mart wardrobe.

"It's just hard to look at anything else," says Nance Mitchell, a licensed aesthetician who waxes away the extra hair of high-profile clients in Beverly Hills. "A man can be talking about business, and all the other person is thinking about is his nose hair."

Not a pretty picture. It seems a cruel twist of fate that just as we lose hair from atop our heads, we start sprouting it from embarrassing places such as our nose and ears. Why does it happen?

"It's a hereditary thing," says Allan Kayne, M.D., assistant clinical professor of dermatology at the University of Washington in Seattle. "You can look to your father and grandfather to see the pattern of hair growth in your family, but there's no truth to the myth that people who lose hair on their heads start to grow hair out of their ears, nose, or other body parts. One thing has nothing to do with the other." In other words, your body's not confused or cruel, it's just one of the changes that accompanies aging.

And it's not always Mother Nature who bestows the gift of hair. Some medications that men take as they get older can change the amount of hair on their bodies. "Any kind of hormonal supplementation, such as Proscar, which fights prostate enlargement, can promote hair growth," explains Toby Zachian, M.D., clinical assistant professor of dermatology at Thomas Jefferson University Hospital in Philadelphia. "Unfortunately, though, we can't yet specify where we want the hair to grow."

The Long and Short of It

Let's face it, it's not the biology of excess body hair that's disturbing; it's the aesthetics. "Hair coming over the collar of a business shirt or growing out of your nose and ears is just unkempt-looking," Mitchell says. "Men remove extra hair to improve their business persona as well as to make a good impression with their friends and the women in their life."

Which begs the question: How much hair is too much? It's really a matter of personal preference. While few of us (men or women) want to see ear hair, not all of us are bugged by excess back or chest hair.

"I don't think that back hair bothers most men," says Philip Kingsley, a hairdresser in London and New York City, and author of *Hair: An Owner's Handbook*. "We generally consider it to be a sign of virility. In fact, I've seen thousands of clients, and not one has ever complained about their body hair." But, as Kingsley concedes, it's not something he would talk about anyhow.

If you do want to get rid of unsightly body hair, Dr. Kayne says it's important to understand this: There's no such thing as permanent hair removal. During electrolysis, for example, an electric charge is sent into the follicle, so that the eventual scarring will render the hair incapable of growing. But it can take multiple visits to induce the proper scar, says Dr. Kayne, and that's only for a small patch of hair.

That said, there are effective ways to keep body hair

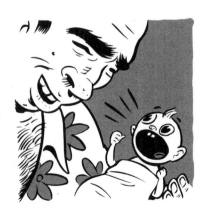

under control. Here are the two best, recommended by our experts.

Get in fighting trim. "Whatever you do, don't try to cut it with any sort of scissors, especially on your own. You'll cut yourself, no question about it," says Dr. Kayne. "Without a doubt, your best option is to use electric snippers or razors, especially those made for the ears and nose." Likewise, a hair stylist, who may or may not take an electric razor to your ears as part of her service, should never use scissors, because if she cuts you, there is, as Dr. Kayne says, "public blood around."

While there are alternatives to nose and ear hair trimmers, you should know that they are painful, dangerous, and a lot more expensive.

You can buy trimmers for both ear and nose hair at a drugstore or through upscale catalogs, such as The Sharper Image. Manufactured by Panasonic, Conair, and other personal-grooming electronic companies, the trimmers are priced anywhere from $12.99 to $32. They run on batteries and are wet/dry, which means that you can rinse them off in a basin full of water.

Taking only a few seconds, the trimmers simply whir around your ears or nostrils, removing just enough hair to neaten you up. There's no way to tell how often you'll need to clip, because that depends on hair growth, but trimming the hair won't make it grow back any faster, longer, or thicker.

Don't be browbeaten. If you aim for that gruff look, then bushy eyebrows are for you. If not, you'll probably want to do some cleaning up. Your options here include tweezing and waxing. Never shave your eyebrows, Mitchell says, because stubble doesn't belong anywhere other than your cheeks. There's also a good chance that you'll go overboard and end up with less eyebrow

Wax and Wane

There are actually men who pay money to have melted wax dripped onto their skin and then yanked off. Think giant Band-Aid.

"I have swimmers, bodybuilders, actors, and bicyclists come in for various waxings," says Nance Mitchell, a licensed aesthetician in Beverly Hills who has performed what she calls a tri-waxing—which includes waxing nose, ear, and back hair—on numerous clients. Since many of her clients are on the big screen, they may need those extra precautions, because one long nose hair could show up as the size of a shoelace.

But that's not an issue for most of us. And neither is waxing, says Chérie M. Ditre, M.D., clinical assistant professor of dermatology at Allegheny University Hospital School of Medicine, Hahnemann Division, in Philadelphia and a former cosmetologist. "I strongly advise against waxing ear and nose hair," Dr. Ditre says. "Those hairs provide a filtration system against infection, and you risk getting a staph infection from total removal."

than you bargained for, and no eyebrow is not a look for anyone.

If you want to tweeze yourself, the key, says Mitchell, is to pluck only about a finger's-width of hair between your eyebrows and just the longest, most straggly hairs from the actual brow. Check out the medicine cabinet of close women friends—chances are that you'll find angled tweezers (they grasp the hair more easily). They also can be bought in the nail-care section of a drugstore.

And don't forget to use the two-mirror approach. Magnify for the actual tweezing, but keep switching to a regular view to make sure that you're not taking too much off. The pain factor is minimal for most people.

Hands

Getting a Grip on Good Grooming

A manicure is one of the cheaper frivolities in a woman's life (on average they cost $12 to $20 for both sexes). Most men don't feel comfortable handing over their fingers to a stranger. Which is fine. A man can still strike a balance between coarse, dry hands and baby's-bottom-soft hands without turning to professionals. Hand and nail care is easy, and it has very tangible benefits.

"Well-groomed hands always make a nice impression, not only in social situations but also in business," says Danielle Korwin, owner of Parts Models in New York City. "It's something that a man shouldn't neglect. Nails should show just a little bit of the white. And since there's nothing worse than ragged cuticles, a man should take the time to push them back."

For the Want of a Nail

Although you'll probably be taking care of your own hands, it's helpful to understand the steps that compose a traditional manicure. "The first thing that I do is clip a man's nails," says Firozé, a manicurist and pedicurist in New York City. "I file them, put cream on their hands, and give them a massage, focusing on certain pressure points to help relax them. Then they soak their hands in warm, soapy water to soften the skin. Finally, I push back their cuticles." Firozé adds that while some guys like the buffed look for nails, for the most part, natural is better.

To care for your own nails, get one of those small nail clippers that are available at all drugstores and newsstands. Here's what to do with them.

Use several small clips per nail. "Turn your hand around so that it's facing you and the tips of your nails are pointing down," advises Firozé. "This gives you the best view." As for clipping, don't start at the sides; rather, clip your way down from the center of the nail. Clip the sides of the nails only after you have flattened the top off to the appropriate length. This will prevent tears or odd-shaped curves. Don't cut your whole nail at once, because that will bend the nail and put too much pressure on the nail bed, which can lead to permanent damage.

Smooth them down. Use a "block" file, which can be found in drugstores, to smooth your newly cut edges. A block file is a white cube of foam that has file paper wrapped around it; it's easier and less effeminate for a guy to use.

File your nails in one direction to reduce the chance of splitting the nail. It is okay to round the corners a bit, but don't file the sides of your nails, advises Firozé. That weakens the edges and causes them to break. Remember that you're only using the file to clean up the trim, not to reduce the size of your nail. If there's a lot of removal to be done, go back to clipping.

Stay away, too, from fine-tuning with the metal file that comes with your nail clipper. These are too rough and will split your nail. So what's that thing for anyway? "It's great for cleaning under your nail," Firozé says. "Just

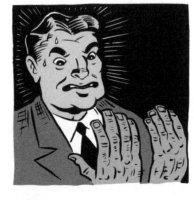

don't go too far in, because you can cut yourself." And by the way, cleaning should be done before cutting.

Clip in private. What's the biggest sin committed during nail care? Clipping your nails in front of people. An economist that we know asked his wife's permission to kill anyone who clipped their fingernails on the subway. She gave it to him.

Justifiable homicide.

Tend to your cuticles. A cuticle is that somewhat hard piece of skin surrounding the bottom of your nail. When uncared for, dead skin cells accumulate under them, leading to a raggedy, dry appearance, Firozé says. If you keep cuticles moist with lotion and push them back, they remain virtually unnoticeable, which should be your ultimate nail goal.

While women usually wrap cotton around an orange stick (basically just a thin, round piece of wood that slants on one end) to push back their cuticles, you don't have to get that fancy. "One of the best ways to take care of your cuticles is to push them back with a washcloth or towel after your shower," suggests Firozé.

Don't push cuticles back with your other fingernails, an X-Acto knife, pen, keys, or any other instrument, because they put too much pressure on your nail bed and can actually change the shape of the nail forever, Firozé cautions. Cutting your cuticles also is not necessary and can lead to those little cuts often seen around a guy's finger. Cuticles are there to protect the nail, so complete removal isn't what you're going for, Firozé says.

Grease: Glove at First Sight

While a little grease is sexy, a lot of grease is poisonous. So if you're going to work on your car or any other piece of machinery, do yourself—and anyone else you're going to touch—a favor and wear gloves. "We started wearing gloves about five years ago," says Patrick Cadam, a mechanic and owner of Pat's Garage in San Francisco.

"First, because petroleum is a hazardous chemical, and second, the solvents that we used to get it off our hands took all the oil out of our skin. It's like washing your hands in paint thinner."

So Cadam borrowed surgical gloves from his wife, a nurse, and found that since wearing them didn't interfere with his dexterity around the engine, it paid to keep his paws covered. "It's not a guy thing to do," says Cadam, "but it's almost as if I didn't work on cars. And the truth is that the rest of life is going to give you calluses anyway, so you might as well take care of your hands when you can.

"I do get careless about it, but after a few days without gloves, my hands look like hell again and then I just end up putting them back on. It's an instant reminder."

Handy Hints

Walk into your local drugstore and you could drop a small fortune buying lotions, potions, and ointments for each body part. Or you could just get a big bottle of unscented Jergens or Lubriderm or any of the big-name, all-purpose skin lotions. Chances are that it will serve your needs. And what are your needs? A few drops on your hands in the morning after a shower, rubbed well in on both sides. That's all that's required to keep your hands soft enough to hold your partner's hand with confidence, says Firozé. "It's no big deal," she adds. Exactly.

Remember that your hands should be slightly moist when you put lotion on. The point isn't to use the lotion to add moisture to your hands but rather to trap moisture in.

Finally, here are a few more thoughts on hand care.

Along with lotion, you should always keep nail polish remover around. No, you're not going to be removing nail polish, but the stuff will clean up lots of other things, including glue, paint, and hair dye. Always keep a bottle around. It's toxic and helpful. Look for remover without formaldehyde, since that's the poison ingredient that can lead to allergic rashes.

Feet

It Takes a Tough Man to Make a Tenderfoot

Taking care of your feet may seem like an act of vanity, but in reality, it's just preventive medicine. Our feet carry the weight of our world, and that can be a heavy load to bear. How heavy? In an average day, your feet absorb 5.7 million pounds of pressure. Although men wear more comfortable shoes than women (even our sneakers and loafers tend to fit better), unlike women, most wouldn't be caught dead getting a pedicure or taking the time to give themselves the at-home alternative.

"Men don't make foot care a part of their daily routine," says pedicurist Firozé, who keeps male models' feet attractive. "That's why they end up having more serious problems, such as calloused skin on their heels and ingrown toenails."

To keep your feet in great shape, all you need are three things: a pumice stone, nail clippers, and moisturizer. And you'd better believe that the little amount of work that you do today will pay off when your toes wander over to the other side of the bed. Here's how to toe the line.

Get a piece of the rock. If you're a little nervous about this pedicure thing, consider this: What could be more manly than scraping off dead skin with a rock? That's precisely what you need the pumice stone for. If you've never taken good care of your feet, there's probably a few years' worth of dead skin encrusted on your heels. A pumice stone is—and looks like—a piece of volcanic rock with lots of air pockets in it. It's

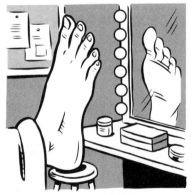

very lightweight, and when rubbed against your foot, it will remove the top layer of skin.

"Men should always have a pumice stone in their shower that they use on a daily basis," says Firozé. While you won't be able to remove a year's worth of dead skin in one session, you'll see a difference in a week or two.

Go in for an oil change. "The reason why we have so much dry skin on our feet is because they get moist in our shoes all day and then dry out too quickly when we go home and take our shoes off," explains William J. Sarchino, D.P.M., president of the medical staff of Mary McClellan Hospital in Cambridge, New York. "It would be much more beneficial to change to a clean pair of socks than go barefoot."

To combat dry skin, always moisturize your feet right after coming out of a bath or shower. "This is also true if you soak your feet," says Dr. Sarchino. "Moisturizing afterward will really keep them soft." While sweat dries out the skin, lotion mixed with the water keeps the skin hydrated.

Firozé believes that the extreme low-fat diets that some people follow can rob skin of needed moisture and nutrients, so she recommends that her clients with dry skin increase the amount of olive oil and avocados that they eat. "They are natural sources of fat and will help keep your heels from cracking," she says.

Dr. Sarchino thinks that it's worth a try, although, he adds, "you don't want to eat just any kind of fat. Stick to small amounts of natural oils rather than high-fat processed food."

File them away. The final—and easiest—step to ensuring that you're on a good foundation is well-trimmed nails. "Always cut your toenails straight across," says Dr. Sarchino. "Don't cut the corners, since that will lead to ingrown toenails." Cutting Vs, or any other shape into the nail, will not guard against ingrown toenails.

If the edges of your nails are jagged after cutting, use a nail file to smooth them, but never use the metal file encased in your nail clipper. It's too rough and will cause the nail to split, advises Firozé. Instead, you'll have to rely on a "block" file, a white cube of foam that has file paper wrapped around it. You can buy a block file in the nail-care section of the drugstore.

Children of the Corn

When it comes to shoes, there is one simple rule of thumb—or toe, as the case may be—that takes precedence over any issue of price or style: If it doesn't fit, you must not buy it. If you do, you'll get more than you bargained for, namely corns, calluses, bunions, and blisters. These unattractive manifestations form when a poorly fitted shoe causes friction against your foot, says Dr. Sarchino. What type of buildup you end up with depends on genetics or where the shoe rubs your foot. Bunions, for example, run in the family.

Calluses are buildups of dead, yellowish skin that usually form on the bottom of your feet to protect the skin, bones, and muscles from further abrasion. Blisters form when the outer layer of skin separates from the lower layer and liquid fills the space in-between.

If callous buildup occurs on your toes (and its growth runs rampant), then the dead skin turns into a corn. Similarly, bunions form on the toes when the friction from tight shoes incites bone growth in and around the joints.

Breathe a Sigh of Relief

If you're not taking proper care of your feet, you'll know it—when you inhale. And so will everyone else within whiffing distance. Odor-causing bacteria thrive in warm, moist environments—like your socks and shoes.

"It's a sign of hyperhydrosis, or sweating of the feet," says Dr. William J. Sarchino of Mary McClellan Hospital. So fight the moisture, and chances are that you'll kill foot odor, too.

The first step is to make sure that your shoes are made of natural, rather than synthetic, materials. Look for as much leather as possible, or canvas if you're buying knockabout sneakers. "The same goes for socks," says Dr. Sarchino. "Stay away from nylon and other materials that increase heat." Cotton is a better choice, he says.

Changing your shoes every day and airing them out on a wooden shoe rack will allow them to dry between wearings, which will cut down on moisture, advises Dr. Sarchino. Powder and charcoal inserts are designed to decrease moisture, and they may help, too.

Another problem associated with moisture and heat is athlete's foot. You'll know you have it if your feet burn, itch, and look dry and scaly. "Athlete's foot is a fungus, and feet trapped in shoes all day are a perfect place for it to grow," explains Dr. Sarchino. "You can try over-the-counter products, and if that doesn't work, see a doctor." To avoid it, wear rubber sandals in the shower, especially in public locker rooms.

Finally, wash your feet daily. "It's not good enough to simply let the water swish around your feet, either," Dr. Sarchino says. "Use your hands or a washcloth to wash your feet and between your toes, and then dry those areas, too."

Skin Care

Getting Below the Surface

For a long time, it seems, men took the statement that "beauty is only skin deep" to mean they needn't muss and fuss over something as superficial as skin care.

"There's no argument that men traditionally were reluctant to buy grooming products," says William Lauder, president of Origins Natural Resources, a subsidiary of Estée Lauder Companies that makes skin care products. "It took them a while to get over the self-consciousness of buying self-care products in the same way women have been doing for a long time. But once they realized that grooming could be a fun—not a tedious—chore that, by the way, made them look and feel great, they jumped on the bandwagon."

It has taken a bit of savvy marketing, macho names, and rugged guy-oriented packaging—check out Clinique's Scruffing Lotion, Polo Sport's Face Fitness moisturizer, Safari for Men's oatmeal soap, and Origins' Swept Clean "special sloughing" for oily skin—but men have indeed jumped, turning men's grooming products into an industry that some estimate is worth $3.3 billion in sales overall.

No matter how old you are, if you haven't already jumped, put on your parachute and say hello to the squeaky-clean world of men's skin care.

About Face

"A man's face is his business card today," says Uri Ben-Ari, president of Jeunesse Cosmetics, a company that markets skin care products

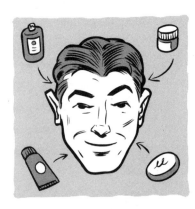

containing minerals from Israel's Dead Sea. "It's what they see first, what they judge you by first, and what they remember last—hopefully it's a good memory."

It's also a dependable timetable of a man's life, says Dr. Seth L. Matarasso of the University of California at San Francisco. Here he itemizes what to expect at each decade and offers some quick solutions.

The Twenties

Problems: Not many unless—like every other self-conscious young man—you consider oiliness and acne serious problems. Meanwhile, by your late twenties, collagen, the substance that helps skin maintain its elasticity, begins decreasing by about 1 percent a year (especially in areas exposed to the sun).

Solutions: "This is basically a maintenance and prevention age," says Dr. Matarasso. "You're insuring against problems that will crop up later." On your face, use mild soaps that are glycerin-based, nonabrasive, and nonirritating (he recommends Dove, Neutrogena, Purpose, and Basis). He also advises using soaps that are "allergy-tested" and "fragrance-free." That means no smelly chemicals added. Soaps like Irish Spring contain deodorants and antibacterial chemicals, making them good shower soaps to wash your hairy parts—underarms, groin, buttocks—but bad for the sensitive face area.

To help prevent acne, he recommends alcohol-based topical antibiotics (Cleocin-T and Erycette) or benzoyl peroxide products available over the counter. Rather than pimple creams like Clearasil, he suggests a light astringent (a drying agent that removes surface debris and whose active ingredient is usually alcohol, witch hazel, or propenyl glycol). For acne blemishes, he recommends Retin-A, a prescription cream containing Vitamin A,

Tattoo You?

Some say it's self-mutilation. Others call it art. But one thing is certain: Tattoos and piercings are on the rise. According to one survey at the beginning of the 1990s, 5 percent of the male population had a tattoo. Estimates of men who have had parts of their bodies pierced are harder to come by, although Dennis Rodman alone would hopelessly skew any average anyway.

"The demographics of people who get pierced started changing in the 1980s," says Michaela Grey, chairwoman of the Association of Professional Piercers and founder and director of training seminars for Gauntlet International, a San Francisco–based piercing business with locations in Los Angeles, Paris, Seattle, and New York City. "They were lawyers, professors, and doctors. The street people certainly couldn't afford $100 a pop."

Getting in Touch

Tattooing, piercing, and other forms of body adornment have been how one tribe distinguishes itself from another—for religious, artistic, political, and sexual reasons—since prehistoric times. These days they may be "one way to get back in touch with our own humanity in an increasingly technological age," Grey theorizes. "The pain they inflict puts you back in touch with your body."

With tattooing, you're creating microscopic punctures in the skin. Expect some bleeding and about a week to heal. Piercing is a puncture wound. Some areas—the tongue or the penis—heal within weeks. Others—nipples, the navel, ears, and nose—can take months. Performed incorrectly or with unsterile equipment, either procedure could result in a very nasty infection.

If you decide a skull-and-crossbones tattoo or gold ring piercing some public or private part of your body adds to your appeal, make your personal health—not your personal artistic statement—your primary concern, suggests Whitney D. Tope, M.D., assistant professor in the Department of Dermatology at the University of Minnesota Medical School in Minneapolis.

"For both piercing and tattooing, safety should come before style," he says. "Make sure they use sterilized tools and other single-use materials to prevent the transmission of blood-born pathogens like hepatitis B and C and HIV, the virus that leads to AIDS."

"This should not be an impulse decision," Grey agrees. "Do your homework. Check out the reputations of piercers and tattooists by talking with previous clients. Ask to see their equipment. Get a feel. Trust your intuition." You have little else to go on: There is no certification for piercing, says Dr. Tope. However, tattooing is licensed by some states and cities.

If you wake up the next morning and realize the tattoo of Mother Teresa on your chest may put off your own mother, a technique called infrared coagulation will erase the mistake—for about $250 (if you don't mind a small scar) and about $750 (if you want to remain scarless).

which also does wonders for wrinkles. To ward off the effects of the sun, get into the habit now of using a sunscreen with a sun protection factor (SPF) of at least 15 (for a detailed explanation of sunscreen, see below).

The Thirties

Problems: First signs of crow's-feet around the eyes. If you haven't been using sunscreen, wrinkles start to show. Elasticity keeps stretching the skin; eyelids begin to droop. Little brown freckles (called solar lentigines) begin to surface. Blood vessels may appear on the top layer of skin. Skin becomes duller looking.

Solutions: Slap on that sunscreen (increase from 15 to 20 or 30 SPF, depending on your sensitivity); it may help reverse early damage. And return to that Retin-A to remove the dead outer layer of skin. "This will slowly get rid of discolorations like brown spots, and it helps improve and prevent fine lines," Dr. Matarasso says.

There is a popular myth that moisturizers get rid of wrinkles. They don't, according to Dr. Matarasso. They just fill in and hydrate the wrinkle—a deft camouflage technique women have long known.

And here's an inside scoop: AHA has become *the* acronym of anti-aging agents. Researchers found that after 22 weeks of twice-daily use of creams containing alpha hydroxy acids (AHAs), 70 percent of users noticed overall improvement on their face and significant reduction in roughness on their arms. Look for face moisturizing creams containing 8 percent glycolic acid or 8 percent lactic acid.

The Forties

Problems: Sleep lines—deep ravines—form in the forehead. The lines at the corners of

---

We All Shine On

You say you walked into a wall. He says you walked into his fist. Why squabble over facts? Your pride may be bruised, but not as badly as that black eye you're sporting. Try these to save face fast.

Chill out. A cold compress will decrease blood flow and reduce swelling. Rather than smashing ice into a towel, use a plastic bag of frozen vegetables. You weren't planning to eat them anyway. Try to keep it on your eye for 20 minutes, then give it a 10-minute break. Repeat over a three-day period or until you're ready to go another few rounds.

Go tropical. Eat fruits—especially tropical fruits like pineapple and papaya, which contain enzymes that help tissues absorb blood more easily. That will fade the black and

---

the nose and mouth—called nasolabial folds—may begin to resemble the Grand Canyon. Those brown sun freckles mushroom like . . . mushrooms. Skin gets drier and even more elastic. Double chin may appear.

Solutions: Continue to religiously apply the moisturizer and sunscreen. To combat facial wrinkles, sleep on your back (practice breathing through your mouth so that you don't snore). Maintain body weight. If you yo-yo diet, the skin will stretch to accommodate your heavier weight, but it doesn't always return to its previous state when you drop those pounds.

The Fifties and Beyond

Problems: Oil gland activity slows down, making your skin dry and flaky. You lose skin pigment. Once-tiny sun and age spots now look like lunar craters. Wrinkles increase, especially around the mouth. Lips get thin, the tip of your nose will droop, and you'll form

blue colors ringing your eye. **Papaya in capsule form (600 milligrams four times a day) will also do the trick.**

Take C and see. Vitamin C promotes healing. Pop a C tablet or down it naturally by eating more broccoli, mangoes, peppers, sweet potatoes, and oranges.

Avoid aspirin. Aspirin prevents blood from clotting, and it's the seepage of blood that leads to discoloration. If you're in pain, reach instead for Tylenol (or any other pain reliever containing acetaminophen).

Cover it up. When all else fails, and you have to go public with your mug, pick up Dermablend at a pharmacy. It's a makeup product that hides skin discoloration caused by broken blood vessels, says Dr. Seth L. Matarasso of the University of California at San Francisco.

jowls. What are jowls? Think Richard Nixon. Medically speaking, it's when the masseter muscles around your jaws get thicker, a localized accumulation of fat similar to the syndrome women deal with in other parts of their bodies as they age. Who gets jowls? Men whose fathers had them. "It's genetic," says Dr. Matarasso. "Beyond that, the culprit is gravity. It pulls you down with age."

Solutions: Same drill as before. Since loss of pigment means loss of skin protection, sunscreen is more critical than ever. If your thin lips bug you, grow a mustache. To remove sun and age spots, you can undergo cryosurgery (liquid nitrogen) or buy a bleaching cream.

The Sun Sets on Suntans

The actor George Hamilton is remembered less for the roles that he played than the tan that he displayed. But by the 1990s, as the evidence linking exposure to the sun and skin cancer mounted, even Hamilton began to turn a lighter shade of pale.

For the fair-skinned, it is that ultraviolet (UV) radiation from the sun that turns you a vibrant shade of lobster. Long-term, even those who attain that Hollywood-style tan pay in skin blemishes, skin that prematurely reminds you of raisins, cataracts and other eye ailments, and skin cancer, of which melanoma is the most serious type.

The Food and Drug Administration (FDA), in conjunction with several skin care and cancer organizations, offers the following seven steps you can take immediately to stage a counterattack on the sun.

1. The easiest way to dodge the sun's UV rays is to stay in the shade, especially from 10:00 A.M. to 3:00 P.M., when the sun's rays are strongest.

FYI: Clouds block only 20 percent of UV radiation. Also, being in a pool or in the ocean is no safeguard; UV radiation passes through water.

Get UV forecasts from the National Weather Service daily within a 30-mile radius of about 60 American cities. Phone companies, newspapers, and TV and radio stations often broadcast UV indexes.

2. Intellectually, you know that it's a no-brainer: Put on the sunscreen. But practically, you have to baste yourself with this smelly, oily, sticky stuff, and you think you look so corny doing it.

Forget the self-consciousness and the inconvenience. Your skin will thank you years from now. The FDA requires all sunscreen and sunblock products to state their sun protection factor. Depending on your sunburn and tanning history, the FDA recommends the following SPF levels.

Lose That Excess Baggage

The eyes are the windows of the soul, some hopeless romantic once said. (And shameless guys have used it as an opening line ever since.) It's too bad when heavy bags make those baby blues look like they've been through the dark night of the soul. Here are some ways to unload some of that luggage.

Try tea for two. Place two moist tea bags over your closed eyes for 15 minutes. The tannin in the tea leaves helps pull the skin taut and reduces puffiness. The cold reduces swelling.

Nuke it with a cuke. Take the same approach as with the tea bags, only use two slices of chilled cucumber.

- Level 2 to under 4 if you rarely burn and tan naturally
- Level 4 to under 8 if you burn minimally, always tan well
- Level 8 to under 12 if you burn moderately and tan gradually
- Level 12 to under 20 if you always burn easily and tan minimally
- Level 20 to 30 if you always burn easily and rarely tan

3. Go under cover. Here's your chance to play Harrison Ford as Indiana Jones. Wear a hat with a brim about three inches wide to cover your neck, ears, nose, eyes, and scalp. Though it won't guard your neck or ears, a baseball cap saves your nose—providing you wear the brim in the front.

4. Here's one more excuse to exude that suave who's-that-famous-guy-behind-the-shades look. Sunglasses with lenses that have UV protection will guard your eyes from sun damage. Dark-tinted shades don't necessarily have more protection—or any protection at all. The best are large-framed wraparounds to keep the sun from sneaking round the corners.

5. Wear sun-blocking clothes. There's more protection wearing thicker fabrics, tighter weaves, and darker colors. Wet clothing won't block UV rays.

Several companies are now marketing clothing they claim offers SPF levels of 30 or more. For example, Solumbra from Sun Precautions (based in Everett, Washington) has received FDA clearance to market its clothing at the SPF level of 30.

Meanwhile, in 1995 the FDA turned over regulation of this sort of apparel to the Consumer Protection Safety Commission (CPSC), an independent Federal agency responsible for the safety of home products. It established a subcommittee to determine which clothing manufacturers are pulling the UV wool over the public's eyes and which are for real, according to Ken Giles, a CPSC spokesman.

6. FDA scientists found that people who use sunlamps 100 times a year may be increasing their exposure to "melanoma-inducing" radiation by 24 times. With all the warnings the FDA includes for artificial tanning devices, the wise consumer would beware—and be fair (skinned, that is). Just say no to tanning lamps.

7. Periodically, give your whole epidermal layer—all 20 square feet of it—a thorough once-over. Use a hand mirror to examine your body for spots after you've showered. Keep an eye on things if they change—like changes in size, texture, shape, and color of moles, freckles, and other discolored patches. A sore that doesn't heal is a warning as well. If you see something developing over time, don't play Russian roulette with your skin: See a dermatologist.

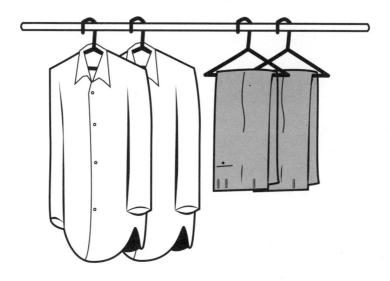

Part Three

Fashion

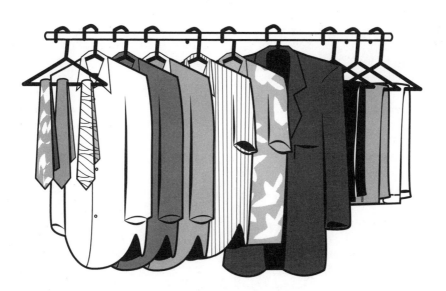

Fashion Sense

Developing a No-Nonsense Approach

What do they take us for? Shills? Lemmings? Pawns? Puppets? As much as it sometimes tries, the fashion industry cannot herd men into conformity and bad taste as it does twice a year to women with its spring and fall lines.

Certainly, it has tried. Shall we count the ways? Leisure suits. Nehru jackets. Double-breasted shirts. Yellow golf pants. Velour warm-up suits, for gosh sakes. And remember this thankfully short-lived fad: the dickey, false turtlenecks that ended at our shoulders?

But we have resisted. Mostly. Okay, maybe we've slipped from time to time, succumbed to such silliness as leather vests with long fringes or Earth shoes. But for the most part, men have held the line. Sometimes, perhaps, to a fault. "Changes in men's fashions can be measured in quarter-inches," says menswear fashion designer Alfred Arena, chairman of the menswear department at the Fashion Institute of Technology in New York City. "I have noticed through the years that men lean toward the traditional look. Younger men are more adventuresome, more willing to take chances and try different looks. But the older a man gets, the more he conforms to what he thinks are the requirements. It's unfortunate because we tend to lose our individuality."

"It amuses me when I hear people say that men are boring dressers," says H. Kristina Haugland, assistant curator of costumes and textiles at the Philadelphia Museum of Art. From the earliest times, men were as much the fancy Dans as were their Dianas. That is, until that dark period in men's fashion known as the Great Renunciation of the late eighteenth and early nineteenth centuries. This coincided with the Industrial Revolution, when men had to punch time clocks, not powder their noses. Those long, fancifully embroidered silk frocks just didn't cut it anymore on the assembly line. Exit self-expression. Enter boredom. Quickly followed by the gray flannel suit.

The Clotheshorse and Other Stallions of Style

The Greek philosopher Epictetus said it better than Calvin Klein ever could: "Know, first, who you are, and then adorn yourself accordingly."

We'll restate and elaborate: When it comes to clothes, having maximum style means, first, having a clear sense of how you want to appear and, second, knowing how to achieve that appearance. Implicit in the second part is having at least some appreciation for the art of clothing. It means being aware that some fabrics are nicer than others; that some colors whisper, while other colors shout; that there is a difference in quality between $20 and $60 pants (and knowing what the difference is); that nice

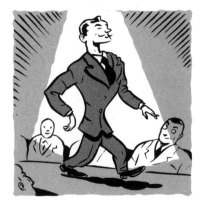

shoes always make a good impression. It means that you are observant of—not obsessed with—how people around you dress and what currently is being touted at your local men's store.

"Your clothes are an extension of yourself," says image consultant Ann Frees, vice-president of Harmony, an organizational management firm in Bethesda, Maryland. That means that every time you get dressed, she suggests, ask yourself at least some of the following questions.

- What do I value?
- What is my vision?
- What are my strengths, my limitations?
- How can I highlight my strengths and make my limits work to my benefit?
- What do I want my appearance to say about me?
- What do I wear to answer all of the above?

That's a lot of heavy-duty introspection before your first cup of coffee. But how you answer them could determine how the rest of your day—perhaps the rest of your life—could go.

Making Sense

Some guys are slobs. Some guys are total slaves to fashion. In between are the rest of us who just need a little fashion sense knocked into us. Here it is (without the bruises to our wallet).

Focus on fabrics. "Materials are the anchor of style," says Murray Pearlstein, owner of Louis, Boston, an upscale men's and women's clothier. "Designers and stylists begin with the fabric. Build the foundations of your image on them and you can't go wrong." His favorite fabric is saxony. It's a wool weave, more rugged than flannel, less coarse than tweed. "It has the feel of a baby's cheek," he says. "It immediately says: Here is a man who knows style."

Go for the good stuff. Or, as Carolyn Gustafson, a New York City–based image consultant who has appeared on numerous television programs, including *Oprah*, puts it: "Buy quality, buy quality, buy quality." Her rationale for breaking open the piggy bank on a few expensive articles of clothing as opposed to a lot of inexpensive rags is that "it's more important

to look good every day than different every day." If you're a penny-pincher, she suggests that rather than have a heart attack when you get a gander at the price tag of an expensive item, convert it via the cost-per-wear formula. Divide the cost by the number of times that you'll wear it during the life of the garment. And remember, she adds, the better the quality of the garment, the larger the number of wears and the cheaper the cost to wear it each time.

Sweat the small stuff. "The devil is in the details," reminds Pearlstein. Since so little changes in men's fashions from year to year, the way to distinguish yourself is in the minutia. Take color: An average guy will wear a tan shirt. Instead, look for a unique coffee or mocha color. (They have the added advantage of covering coffee and mocha drink stains better.) Reach for unexpected juxtapositions and unpredictable color matches, like that mocha shirt with a burgundy tie. "While nothing seems to go together, it all goes together," Pearlstein says. "People will stop and look and comment on your attractive appearance, but they won't know exactly why."

Buy for feeling, not for status. Buying clothes to impress other people "is the wrong reason," says Pearlstein. "The right reason is to feel good—to feel special. You work better and you think better when you're feeling good about yourself." And clothes can go a long way to getting you into that frame of mind.

Shine with good shoes. Your father was right: You can read much about a man by the shoes he wears. How do *you* want to be read? You could take a chance and wear bright green basketball shoes to work, in the hopes that people will read you as creative and nonconformist. But for most of us, the smarter path is more staid: Wear clean, trim, high-quality leather shoes that are comfortable yet elegant. Make that first impression one of dignity.

The Style Test

You've mastered the basics. It's been years—decades, perhaps—since you committed a mortal sin against style. If you came of age in the 1960s, maybe it was a fringe leather vest, a Nehru jacket, or striped bell-bottoms. If you hit your teens in the 1970s, it could have been platform shoes or a lime green leisure suit. It doesn't really matter. The important thing is that you lived to laugh about it.

Ah, but those venial sins—they're another story. Many of the subtleties and nuances of style, you must confess, still escape you. And it's not just fashion sense. For by now, you've learned that style goes deeper than an Italian suit. That style means saying and doing the right thing at the right moment—for the right reason. There's nothing false or insincere about a man with style.

If only there was a finishing school for men, one that you could attend incognito, perhaps. Now there is: this book. But before you move to the next level of style and sophistication, we'd like you to take this little placement test, put together with the help of G. Bruce Boyer, a private and corporate image consultant in Bethlehem, Pennsylvania, and author of *Elegance* and *Eminently Suitable*. Pass it with flying (complementary) colors, and we'll promote you to the postgraduate seminar. Fail and you're doomed to detention with a roomful of overzealous tailors itching to hem your pants too short. So grab a pen and circle your answers. See below to check your style score.

1. The last time you went clothes shopping, you brought:

   a. Swatches of fabric with various patterns and colors that might work with your existing wardrobe

   b. A walletful of credit cards

   c. Your mother

2. When you want to make an impressive fashion statement, you wear:

   a. An outfit that you picked out from a GQ fashion spread

   b. Such a variety of patterns that anyone looking at you from short range would get astigmatism

   c. Clothes that make you feel like a million dollars—whether they cost that or not

3. Your shoe collection includes:

   a. One pair of Italian-made shoes worth $300

   b. At least one pair of shoes that are so comfortable that you feel like you're wearing socks

   c. Sperry Top-Siders, even though you never have nor ever will set foot on a boat

4. On Casual Friday you wear:

   a. The same dress clothes you usually wear because you think that it's just a passing fad

   b. A pair of well-pressed khakis, a pressed denim shirt, and a tie and sport jacket

   c. Jeans and a T-shirt with the Grateful Dead's dancing skeletons logo on it

5. You have a romantic evening planned with your new girlfriend, and you think that this just might be the night. So you open your underwear drawer and put on:

   a. Your saggy white briefs

   b. A pair of silk boxers

   c. Your special bikini-cut briefs with "Home of the Whopper" inscribed on the front

6. According to custom, the bottom button of a vest should not be buttoned:

   a. In deference to some British monarch who forgot to button his and the members of his court who mindlessly followed suit

   b. In honor of the Earl of Button

   c. Because the bottom button is made to accommodate girth

7. Wearing natural fabrics blended with synthetic materials is a sign that you:

a. Know squat about the finer things in life

b. Can't afford the finer things in life

c. Believe that small percentages of man-made fabrics added to cotton and wool make the fabric more wrinkle-resistant and durable

8. When you take the one you love out to celebrate a special occasion, you:

a. Make sure that every detail is arranged well in advance, from concert tickets to restaurant reservations to the string quartet that will serenade her later at home

b. Surprise her by inviting your bowling team to join you for all of the above

c. Show up at her house with a cold pizza and a couple of warm beers the night after the occasion has passed

9. In conversations, you:

a. Speak only when spoken to

b. Listen only long enough to catch the drift of the conversation and then pontificate on a subject with which you are vaguely familiar

c. Listen more than you talk

10. How would you describe yourself?

a. Jack of a couple trades and a darn good faker when it comes to the rest

b. Jack of all trades and master of one

c. Jack the Ripper

11. When you go out for an evening event, you wear:

a. A set of simple gold cuff links that has been in your family for four generations

b. A gold tooth

c. Enough gold jewelry around your neck to sink the Titanic

12. Your idea of well-groomed is:

a. Spraying deodorant in all the critical places

b. Making sure that your dog's hair is not clinging to your pants

c. Nails clipped, hair trimmed, closely shaven, and freshly showered

13. A stylish man has a multitude of interests, so you enjoy an evening that runs the gamut from:

a. Reading Gabriel García Márquez's 100 Years of Solitude to reading the stock listings

b. Surfing from ESPN to the SportsChannel

c. Opera the Lincoln Center to line dancing at the No Bull Bar

14. A fascinating man that you'd love to spend an evening shooting the breeze with:

a. Stephen Hawking

b. Terry Bradshaw

c. Howard Stern

Scoring

Correct answers: 1. a, 2. c, 3. b, 4. b, 5. b, 6. a, 7. c, 8. a, 9. c, 10. b, 11. a, 12. c, 13. c, 14. all correct.

Add up the number of your correct answers.

11 to 14 correct: **Consider yourself in a league with such stylish men as Cary Grant and Fred Astaire.**

6 to 10: **You know what style is but aren't sure how to pull it off. You'd probably feel comfortable in the company of former President Gerald Ford and Conan O'Brien.**

0 to 5: **You're lucky your shoes match. You'd embarrass Larry, Moe, and Curly.**

Acquiring a Feel for Fabrics

Have Style to the Finish

Oddly enough, it's the feel of a fabric rather than its look that can make you look great.

"A well-educated touch is more important than a well-educated eye when it comes to discerning the type and quality of a fabric," says Debbie Gioello, professor and former chairwoman of the fashion design department at the Fashion Institute of Technology in New York City and author of *Understanding Fabrics*. "The truth comes out in the feel."

The Magic Touch

Feel is also called finish, and, says Gioello, there are two kinds. Hard finishes are flat, smooth, and closely woven. "They feel thin and they're durable," she says. Examples include 100 percent wool or blends of wool or cotton and synthetic fabrics. Soft finishes are thicker and bulkier; they look and feel warmer. They trap heat and are better for winter and casual wear. Flannel is a good example of a soft finish. Hard fabrics hold creases better and "always look sharp and well-pressed," Gioello says. "Softer fabrics don't hold creases unless they're fixed with synthetics."

The feel of fabrics is especially important "for the clothing that touches you," notes Alan Flusser, a New York City menswear designer and author of *Style and the Man*. "Therefore, since most men don't wear undershirts anymore, the most important piece of

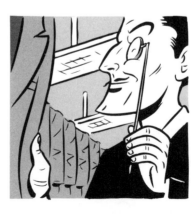

clothing is your shirt." He recommends spending a little bit more for a comfortable cotton shirt, a soft fabric that "breathes."

Short of earning a Ph.D. in textiles or working in a garment factory the rest of your life, here's a quick way to test your touch skill level. Blindfold yourself. Run your fingers across velvet. Now run them across a ripe peach. Now run them across the fabric in question. If you can't tell the difference among the three, the fabric has a high-quality finish and should be part of your wardrobe.

Now that you've let your fingers do the running, here's a rundown of the major fabrics and their qualities.

Cotton

We have Eli Whitney to thank for the comfort of cotton clothing. With the invention of his cotton gin in 1791, cotton replaced wool and linen as king of the textiles. Between 1990 and 1995, U.S. consumer demand for cotton products soared by 42 percent; by 2000, it is expected to jump another 21 percent. Today, cotton covers everything: sweaters, towels, slacks, T-shirts, jeans. You wear it and it's probably made of cotton. You name it and it's probably cotton, too. Among the many names cotton comes in are chambray, chino, corduroy, denim, poplin, seersucker, terry cloth, and velvet.

While comfortable to the touch, one of its most appealing features is that it's hydrophilic. That means that it loves water. Its porous quality absorbs body moisture, keeping your skin dry. That also means that it will wash clean without damaging the fibers.

Cleaning tip. To stretch the life of cotton, always wash it in cold water. Use a small amount of a mild detergent, preferably made with natural or organic ingredients. If it's not sudsing, don't add more soap. ("Read the instructions," advises Claudia Kaneb, wardrobe head for NBC's *Today* and wardrobe supervisor for more than 31 Broadway shows. "It may be low-sudsing.") Put cotton in the dryer for not more than 20 minutes. Use a hot iron. "The less times you have to run the iron over a fabric, the less you beat it up and the longer it will last," she says. While ironing, spray the fabric with water from a plant sprayer or the sprayer on your iron, if it has one.

Wool

Ever since the Stone Age, when early no-mads gathered tufts of fleece that fell from shed-ding sheep and wrapped themselves in it, wool has been softening some of life's harder edges.

Wool works wonders. It resists water but absorbs moisture. It resists wrinkles but can be pressed to hold sharp pleats and folds. It stretches easily but won't sag out of shape. It keeps you warm in cool weather and cool in warm.

Wool is also more flexible than other fab-rics. It will bend up to 20,000 times before it breaks. Cotton breaks after 3,200 bends, silk after 1,800 bends, and rayon after only 75. As a result, you'll find 89 percent of all suits and 74 percent of all sport jackets are either 100 percent wool or wool blends.

What we commonly refer to as wool comes in two types of yarn: woolen and worsted. Woolen yarn is the thicker and more loosely twisted of the two. It's warm and fuzzy, a trait to which many of us aspire. The winter fabrics—flannels, tweeds, and meltons—are all woolen. Worsted yarns are combed to lie parallel to each other, producing a smooth, clean look. They're finer and more tightly twisted than woolen. Gabardines, for example, are worsted fabrics. They're great for moder-ately warm climates and that refined look.

Cleaning tip. Most men would be just as happy to send a woolen sweater to the dry cleaner, "but you'll shorten its life span by sev-eral years," Kaneb says. Wash it in the delicate cycle, using cold water and mild soap. When it's done, "don't ever throw it in the dryer," she warns, or it'll be too small for your kids. Better to lay it flat on a towel on the floor or kitchen table to dry. Flip it over after 12 hours, putting a fresh towel in between. Even better, buy a drying rack to keep air circulating around it.

Synthetics

Called the miracle fiber when it was first introduced in 1951, polyester was one of the first of the man-made or synthetic fabrics (nylon was the first, invented by Du Pont in 1938). It's made by heating two petroleum-based chemicals and forcing the resulting molten liquid through tiny holes to form fibers. If you feel your exposure to petrochemicals should be limited to fill-ups at the gas station, you may not feel comfortable wearing polyester or other synthetics. On the other hand, their utilitarian qualities are hard to beat: wrinkle-resistant, washable/dryable, so long-lasting that they are practically indestructible.

How indestructible? Perhaps the fiber's greatest miracle was surviving—though just barely—the leisure suit craze of the 1970s. Now, thanks to the invention of many new vari-eties, more than 40 percent of all garments made in America contain polyester. In men's apparel alone, 60 percent of dress shirts, 33 per-cent of knit sport shirts, 43 percent of suits, 39 percent of pants, and 78 percent of sleepwear contain polyester.

Among the other brand names that syn-thetics go by are Dacron, Lycra, Coolmax, Sup-plex, Tactel, Thermastat, and Thermax.

"Synthetics are fine for clothing that you don't mind perspiring in," Flusser says. "They aren't made to breathe—and they don't. They're more appropriate for sportswear, though in small percentages they do enhance the performance quality of fabrics like wool."

Cleaning tip. "Polyesters of today are 10 times better than what you may remember from the 1960s and 1970s," says Kaneb. "They wear fairly well." To care for polyester, "pretend that it's a real fabric," she says. The drill is the same: cold-water wash, short dryer cycle, quick iron job. But don't turn your back while you're ironing. You can never tell what the heat will mutate it into.

Detecting a Pattern

Choose Ones That Fit You

Patterns speak volumes about a man, according to Alison Lurie, professor of English at Cornell University in Ithaca, New York, a novelist who became so fascinated with fashion that she wrote an entertaining nonfiction book about it entitled *The Language of Clothes.*

"I have noticed a direct correlation between the size of the patterns that a man tends to wear and the obviousness of his character," she says. "Men who like to wear large-size patterns make large, bold gestures. Men drawn to small, complicated patterns often have intricate, complicated minds. Men who wear thin blue-checked shirts that look like accountants' ledgers are generally subtle, ordered men of detail, men that you can trust keeping your books."

Solids may be a sign of insecurity, Lurie says. Checks and plaids often say conservative. Stripes cover a variety of personality types, from the closet comedian who wears wide ones to the intellectual who thinks thin.

In the old days, when you could actually afford to have those dots and stripes hand-woven into the fabric, patterned clothing meant prestige. Today, it means that you're smart enough to know that all those crosshatches and dots camouflage ink spots and food stains. Seriously, though: Finer, tinier, and more subtle patterns are considered dressier these days. The louder, bigger, and bolder the patterns, the more suitable for casual wear.

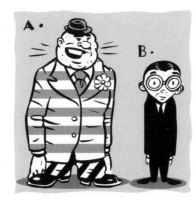

The Big Three

If you want to keep the world guessing your true nature, keep changing your patterns. That shouldn't be hard. There are only three basic choices, with slight variations. They are:

• *Solids.* What's a pattern with no patterns? A solid. Here, the only choice is color. "When in doubt, a solid is the simplest, most effective, and always-acceptable choice," says nationally renowned image expert and syndicated columnist John T. Molloy, author of the bestselling book *John T. Molloy's New Dress for Success.* In other words, it's a safe call. The safest, he recommends, are blue, gray, and beige.

• *Stripes.* Here's the easy part: Stripes are lines that go vertically (very few men look good in stripes that go horizontally). "Vertical stripes definitely make heavy men look thinner and short men look taller," says Jerry Kwaitkowski, executive vice-president of design for Perry Ellis and a guest critic at Parsons School of Design in New York City. Now for the hard part. Stripes come in many shapes and sizes. Just to get you started, for example, there's the traditional stripe, the pinstripe, the chalk stripe, the wide-space chalk stripe, and the British stripe.

• *Plaids/checks.* These are the patterns that give you astigmatism if you stare at them too long. Glen plaid, also called glen check, originated as Scottish clan plaid. It's a boxlike design formed by lines crossing at right angles. Tartan plaids characteristically consist of a series of checks superimposed over each other to form a larger check. Houndstooth is a broken check that resembles a four-pointed star and can come in tiny and giant versions. Tattersall checks are regularly spaced two-colored lines that cross each other like a game of tic-tac-toe.

Other patterns that don't fall neatly into the above categories include paisley, in which hundreds of amoebas appear to be crawling on your tie; herringbone, a military-like design with thread slanting right and left forming chevron patterns; and the ever-popular polka dots which, depending on their size, connote either circus clowns or corporate chief executive officers. (Yeah, we know—sometimes it's tough to tell the difference.)

Mixing and matching patterns is simple math. You start with three patterns (solids, stripes, and plaids/checks). To keep it simple, you add three articles of clothing (jacket or suit, shirt, and tie). Put your calculator away. Take out your swatches.

There are four ways that a man can combine patterns, says Lisa Cunningham, a New York City–based image consultant who teaches at the Fashion Institute of Technology and is a former international board member of the Association of Image Consultants International.

The easiest and most conservative is in three solid colors. "As long as you're not color-blind, you can't go wrong," she adds. To add some flair, make sure that one color jumps out. The others can be your typical navy, gray, or tan.

The next is mixing two solid colors with one pattern. Again, Cunningham adds, be aware of mixing soft and loud colors.

By now you've guessed the third: two patterns and one solid. "This is where some guys need help," Cunningham says. This fine art depends on making sure that the sizes of the two patterns aren't the same and finding at least one that is the same color in both patterns to pull the two together. For example, match the red thread of a pinstripe suit with a red-striped tie. If you use the same two stripe sizes, though, "you get what I call the prison bars effect," says Cunningham. If the checks are the same size, you start to look like graph paper.

Beginners shouldn't try this fourth option at home alone until they've taken an advanced

Going Wild

Even a well-dressed guy can find his clothes going to the dogs—and the fish. Take houndstooth, for example. It's so named because of its broken check pattern. The design of each would-be square is irregular, but each renegade rectangle is uniform in its irregularity. The resulting pattern is said to resemble canine teeth.

Four light and four dark threads—typically black and white—are intertwined to create this checkered pattern, which usually is smaller for men's clothes and larger for women's.

If the thought of wearing a garment with Cujo's fangs makes you rabid, you might prefer something in herringbone. Its name comes from its zigzag pattern, which supposedly resembles the skeleton of a herring. This classic weave was very popular in the 1940s.

What the heck, if you're going to wear a coat that looks like it's from the wild kingdom, you might as well get the real deal. How about sharkskin? Well, no. Sharkskin coats, like houndstooth and herringbone garments, are a twill weave. Men outside the United States know this and have the good sense to call this popular fabric with the dark and light design a pick-and-pick.

fashion workshop. It's mixing three patterns. Gulp! A feat worthy of Chinese acrobats, no? "This is where guys fall apart," Cunningham says. "It takes talent, great skill, and confidence to pull this off. But it makes a very strong, very fashion-forward statement."

If that's the way you see yourself, proceed with caution. The trick is to use two of one pattern and one of another. Two checks (of different sizes) and one stripe. Or two stripes (of different sizes) and one small plaid or check. Easy. Hey, bring on the juggling plates.

Choosing Complementary Colors

Know What Works for You

Think of yourself as a half-painted portrait. The colors already on the canvas are those of your hair, your eyes, and your skin. The clothes that you pick can make you look picture-perfect. Or not.

"Think about balance, think about composition when you pick the colors of the clothes that you wear," says June Roche, corporate fashion director and color forecaster for Milliken and Company, a textile manufacturer based in Spartanburg, South Carolina. "Most men don't have that awareness, and sometimes it's very obvious."

The wrong colors can make a man seem like someone he isn't, she says. For example, a man with fair hair and skin who wears bold colors may end up looking too mousy, while a man with dark features sporting faded and muted colors will appear overly aggressive.

Breaking the Color Code

There are two ways to pick the right color of clothing, suggests Georgette Braadt, an image and communication consultant based in Allentown, Pennsylvania. One is to select colors that complement your natural body coloring. The other is based on what response you want to elicit from people or a particular situation.

In either case, "everything has to work together," says image consultant Carolyn Gustafson. "Complementary colors may not be complimentary to you."

First you have to know what colors work well with the colors of your hair, eyes, and skin. "Men don't buy that winter-spring-summer-fall thing used by women who have their colors done," she says.

Anyway, she adds, "trying to explain colors is like trying to explain nuclear physics in five sentences." To make it a lot simpler, think about the temperature, the depth, and the intensity of color, she suggests.

Temperature means how "warm" or "cool" your skin, eyes, and hair are. Warm tones are more yellow-based; cool tones are blue-based. A quick way to figure out which world you fall into, Gustafson says, is to stand in front of a mirror in daylight and hold up some produce next to your skin (yes, you read this correctly). If you look better next to a raspberry (contains more blue), you're cool. If, on the other hand, you look peachy next to a tomato (more yellow), you're warm.

Depth refers to lightness and darkness of your coloration. Light hair and skin would pair well with powder blue, while dark features match navy blue. Royal blue would work for somewhere in between.

Intensity is how bright or muted the colors are. Men with muted or softer coloring look better in "dusty or hazy" colors that have a touch of gray or are faded. (President Bill Clinton is an example of muted coloring.) Men with

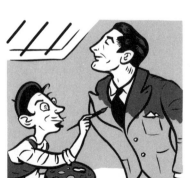

darker complexions and hair look better in bright colors—crisp, clear, rich colors that pop out. (Here's something that you've probably never read before: Sylvester Stallone is bright.) Gustafson offers this white-shirt tip: "Cool" men should wear white shirts. "Warm" men should stick to the ivory or cream variations of white.

The bottom line: "When you wear the colors that are

right for you, you look healthier, more powerful, more energetic," Gustafson says. "The wrong colors can make you look older and sickly, out of sync with yourself."

The Human Coloring Book

"Color has been called the silent salesman and communicates an unspoken message to the consumer at the point of purchase," says Leatrice Eiseman, color specialist and executive director of the Pantone Color Institute in Carlstadt, New Jersey, and author of *Alive with Color*. Here are three things to remember to help paint the impression that you'd like to make *and* help you sell your product.

Take command with high contrasts. Wear a crisp, white shirt and a dark jacket or suit when making a presentation to potential clients. "The high contrast sets off your face and frames you in an authoritative way," Braadt says. Dark sunglasses are powerful and serious. They say that you mean business—on your terms.

Agree to tone it down. If your purpose is consensus, "wear something approachable, in medium softer shades," Braadt says. Powder blues, light greens, and other muted soft shades show off your human side. Their message: You're a team player who can empathize.

Throw a one-two combo to close the deal. Use colors to get what you want. Wear the dark, contrasty, authoritative suit the day that you give the presentation to the client. The next day, when you're trying to get them to sign the contract, switch to the approachable outfit. Once the contract is signed, go home and celebrate in anything you want.

Sending a Message

The right colors also can send subliminal messages. Pantone, the maker of color dyes, in conjunction with Roper/Starch Worldwide Marketing, surveyed men to determine their color preferences and what the colors meant to them. In order of preference, they appear below. And remember, adds Gustafson, when you wear your favorite color, it gives you a certain self-confidence that is almost palpable. Her secret color tip: "Wear colors to match your eye color, and the effect on your overall appearance is magical."

- *Blue.* American men's favorite color, most associated with serenity. Most men prefer the darker shades, between navy and royal blue. The medium shades represent friendship and sincerity; the darker blues, strength and vibrancy.
- *Green.* Ranking second, there are more shades of this than any other color in the spectrum. We shy away from the strong yellow-greens but like the dark forest greens. It symbolizes "new growth and energy and increases your well-being when you wear it," says Roche.
- *Purple.* It nudged out red by a small margin. Considered sophisticated and sexy, purple was once considered too feminine, but the royal purple shades have gained in popularity. It personifies power, royalty, and richness. "Call it grape and men love it," Roche says. "But if you say purple, it still scares off some conservative men."
- *Red.* The survey showed that this was the favorite color of the "most economically secure" white-collar, middle-age achievers who were "unafraid to take risks." Considered the sexiest and most revitalizing color, it represents valor and passion.
- *Charcoal gray and black.* Black embodies power and sophistication. In corporate settings, they're always in style.
- *Brown.* Chosen as the most conservative color, it's also associated with masculine traits.
- *Yellow.* It suggests a man of spontaneity, vivacity, and youth, conveying feelings of fun, warmth, and cheerfulness.
- *Orange.* Unless you're a Hare Krishna, this is men's least favorite, especially bright fluorescent orange. The younger the man, the more he'll wear orange.

Shopping Strategies

How to Get What You Want

Women shop 'til they drop. Men drop at the thought of shopping.

"The average man is very insecure when he goes shopping," says Mortimer Levitt, founder of the Custom Shop men's clothing chain and author of several men's fashion books.

Why? "Either he doesn't know what to buy or he's afraid that the salesman will take advantage of him," suggests Levitt.

There's another reason, adds image consultant G. Bruce Boyer. "He's done so little of it himself," he says. In fact, 52 percent of men say that they don't like to shop for clothes, according to a survey conducted for *DNR (Daily News Record)*, the newsmagazine of men's retail and fashion. And 46 percent say that they like to have someone with them when they shop. In 80 percent of those cases, that someone is a woman.

If you wouldn't send your mother to buy a car for you, why send her or your girlfriend, wife, or daughter to buy something as self-defining as your clothes?

Shopping for Sport

Think of shopping as a competitive event. The better prepared you are, the better you'll do and, incidentally, the more you'll enjoy it. Boyer offers the following tips to lessen the burden of buying.

Make a list. Know what you want and need before you go shopping. Write it down.

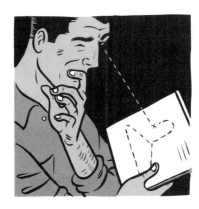

Take that list with you. Don't browse for clothes or impulse-buy. You'll probably end up with things you don't really need that go with nothing else you own—and pay more than you planned to spend.

Let your fingers do the walking. Call around to a variety of stores to ask if they have the item that you're looking for, at what price, and in what colors and sizes. Start with the Yellow Pages or get recommendations from friends for great places to shop. There are now various Web sites and Internet addresses hosted by clothing manufacturers where you can shop by finger.

Bring evidence. If you feel insecure about being able to describe the look that you're after, clip pictures from magazine ads or fashion spreads that come close. Show them to the salesman. If he doesn't sell anything that looks like the pictures that you brought, don't let him steer you toward something else.

Know the sale season. Even though 57 percent of the men surveyed by *DNR* say that "finding a bargain is not as important as finding the right quality," there's no reason that you have to choose one over the other. Sales happen in what the industry calls shoulder seasons. In fashion, that means that you'll find the best buys at the end of January after the holiday rush and in the beginning of August after summer shopping has ended but before fall forays begin.

Ask and ye shall learn. Don't be afraid to ask even the dumbest questions. What is this made of? Wool? Cotton? Blend? What are the buttons made of? Plastic? Ceramic? What are the cleaning instructions? Is there a lining? What type of thread is used? These are the foundations that will begin to educate you as a consumer—and that will help you make wiser buys.

Quit while you're ahead—or behind. Or whenever you have reached your shopping limit. Unlike women, we shouldn't shop 'til we drop. We should shop until we've checked off everything on our list or the thrill is gone.

Shopping Options

The average man shops for clothes less than once a month, or 10½ times a year, according to the *DNR* survey. And the single largest group of men—almost one-quarter of those surveyed—spend between $300 and $499 annually. The biggest clotheshorses live in the city. Urban men spent an average of $707 on new clothes in 1995. Although men in general are spending more on clothes these days—retail sales of men's apparel rose 16 percent from 1991 to 1995, reaching $40 billion—their buying power pales compared to women, who spent $73 billion.

Once you make up your mind to enter the shopping game, you must decide what arena you want to compete in. Leaving out second-hand stores, there are four: the men's department of big stores like Macy's or JCPenney, specialty shops that carry only men's clothing, catalogs, and custom tailors. Here's a rundown of what to expect from them.

Department Stores

Pros: This is where most guys shop. In the *DNR* survey, 46 percent bought their clothes at department stores such as Macy's or Nordstrom; 11 percent shopped at national chains such as Sears; and another 11 percent shopped at discount chains, such as Kmart or Wal-Mart. In general, they offer varieties of styles and probably more choices within each style. Many department stores are designed so that there are stores within stores. One designer may take over a whole corner of the men's section. Another sec-

---

The Tall and the Short of It

We can't all be regular guys. Some of us are extraordinary, at least when it comes to fit. That's where clothing retailers catering to the big guy and the small guy fit in.

At Rochester Big and Tall Clothing, an international chain, the hard part is getting big men to admit that they need an extra large, says Steven Ckolov, vice-president of merchandising for the San Francisco–based company, which dresses men who stand six feet four inches and taller and tip the scales at 200 pounds and up.

The secret of fitting an oversize or undersize man is not in letting it out or taking it in here and there, Ckolov says. It's in proportioning the apparel appropriately. "We design pants, for example, so that a man can wear them where they're intended to be worn, around his waist, as opposed to well below his stomach bulge.

"He can and should wear the newest fashions," says Ckolov. That said, he suggests that big men shy away from bright or wild colors and plaids that have too many vertical or horizontal lines, depending on which way their own lines go.

For the short guy, the basic principles are the same, explains Bob Stern, president and owner of Short Sizes, a national mail-order catalog with a retail store in Cleveland. "It's my goal to dress a man not so that he looks taller but so that he looks his best," says Stern, who stands confidently at five feet two inches. "You can't hide my height. Even if I wore a pinstripe suit with a striped shirt and tie all pointing vertically, I'd still be five feet two inches."

---

tion will be devoted to sportswear or formal wear. Enjoy the three-ring circus atmosphere. Don't rush through the buying experience. Walk around. Take advantage of the crowded floor and ask others' opinions of the item that you've picked out. Also, the price may be somewhat lower. And if you can't find what you want, you can always wander into the hardware department just down the aisle.

Cons: "The guy who's behind the necktie counter this week was selling refrigerators last week, and next week he'll be in the video department," Boyer says. "There's no reason to believe that he has any more knowledge than you about men's clothing." Here's one way to find out. Ask him if the sport jacket that you're looking at is fused or canvas-fronted. Of course, you have to know what that means. Fused means that the manufacturer glued the inner and outer linings together, a less desirable procedure since each dry cleaning will dry the glue a bit. Canvas-fronted is hand-sewn, a more durable method. A good salesman will not only know the difference but also will recommend the canvas-fronted jacket.

Men's Specialty Shops

Pros: "This is my first choice," Boyer says. "I'm the first to admit that I'll pay more, but I look at it this way: If I pay $100 for a jacket that lasts me one year and falls apart, it's more expensive than a jacket I pay $500 for that lasts me 10 years." The best buy in a specialty shop is the store's private label. Get on the store's mailing list for sales available only to regular customers. Also, a regular customer at a specialty store will develop relationships with salesmen who will put aside a shirt for you if they know that you've been looking for one in that style. And alterations are better in specialty stores. The tailor has usually worked there for a while. "Department stores farm out alterations to who knows who?" says Boyer.

Cons: You *will* pay more. Also, your choices will be limited to the tastes of the

---

Star-Crossed Shopping

In your dreams, you're Sean Connery. Or Arnold Schwarzenegger. Or, maybe, even Divine. (Hey, they're your dreams.) Sure, it'll never happen, but—if you have the cash and are willing to part with it—you can at least dress like your favorite celluloid hero, thanks to Norma's Jeans, a celebrity memorabilia mail-order catalog.

The company specializes in clothing and other items once worn, or owned, or at least touched, by the stars. Among the celebrity clothes, costumes, and jewelry that Norma's Jeans has offered are:

- The Army fatigues worn by Tom Hanks in *Forrest Gump* ($20,000)
- The shirt off Robert Redford's back from *Indecent Proposal* ($250)
- An autographed, black bow tie worn by Sean Connery in *Dr. No* ($375)
- The pants Arnold Schwarzenegger wore in *Total Recall* ($595)

---

store's owner. Stores are known for the styles that they prefer. Your selection within each clothing category—jackets, shirts, and so on—may be more limited as well.

Clothing Catalogs

Pros: They began as a utilitarian way for farmers in the boonies to shop the big-city stores without having to drive 200 miles. Now there are catalogs out the wazoo to please any taste, and they're better than ever.

In the old days, it was hard to shop for clothes by mail because the photo reproduction was so bad that the most popular color appeared to be mud. Now, catalogs "are so good that you can almost feel the garment, and descriptions are so detailed and highly technical that you can actually learn something about

- **A red sequined dress worn by Divine, complete with autographed photo of him wearing the dress ($995)**
- **A red paisley vest worn by Jack Nicholson during a scene that eventually wound up on the cutting room floor for *The Witches of Eastwick* ($150)**
- **A jockstrap signed on the front by Madonna ($995)**
- **Shirt collars worn by John Wayne or Boris Karloff ($60)**
- **Shirt collars worn by Steve McQueen or Cary Grant ($45)**
- **Shirt collars worn by Ed Begley, Jr., or James Gleason ($5)**
- **A custom-made two-piece gray wool suit made for Frank Sinatra that Ol' Blue Eyes gave to a friend who wore the same size ($700)**
- **A Marine cap signed by Clint Eastwood and worn by an extra during the filming of *Heartbreak Ridge* ($225)**

For a catalog, send $2 to: Norma's Jeans, 3511 Turner Lane, Chevy Chase, MD 20815-3213. Or phone (301) 652-4644 or fax (301) 907-0216.

how clothes are made," says Susan Ashdown, Ph.D., assistant professor in the Department of Textiles and Apparel at Cornell University in Ithaca, New York.

Men have an advantage over women when it comes to buying apparel through mail-order catalogs, says Dr. Ashdown. For men, what you see is what you get. In other words, a man with a 40-inch chest wears a size 40 jacket. A size 10 dress doesn't mean that a woman has a 10-inch anything.

Cons: Any situation in which you buy something sight unseen—and, in this case, unfelt and unworn—puts you at a disadvantage. They have your money. Period. That's why Dr. Ashdown suggests that you make sure that the return policy is just that: that the company guarantees every item sold (with the general excep-

tion of items that have been monogrammed) and will exchange, substitute, credit, or refund money according to the stipulations in the catalog. If you have any doubts, call the company and ask that the return policy be stated to you. Even with a solid return policy, it can be frustrating and time-consuming to order an item that doesn't fit, send it back, and wait to get another one delivered. And if the truth be known, the photo reproduction could be *National Geographic* quality and you're *still* not going to know what you look like in that alpaca sweater until you try it on.

Custom Tailors

Pros: "Picking a tailor is not unlike picking a doctor," says Suzanne Kilgore, executive director of the Custom Tailors and Designers Association of America, a Washington, D.C., organization. "It's very personal. You should feel like you have the same sense of style." It's also like seeing a doctor when the bill arrives. Anything custom-made for one person tends to cost more than something off the assembly line. But, notes Kilgore, by the time you pay for the alterations for that Armani you bought off the rack, you might be paying the same price as having it custom-tailored. And the Armani still might not fit as though it was made exclusively for your body.

Cons: If you don't like firing your doctor when you're unhappy with the relationship, you're going to feel the same way about firing your tailor—exactly because it is such a personal relationship. If your tailor keeps cutting your jacket in ways that are unflattering for your build, or his sense of style has gone out of style, it's time to part ways. This could be even more sticky if the tailor came by way of recommendation from, say, the person at work who holds your future in his hands.

A Stylish Man's Closet

What You Really Need

Want to really scare yourself? Shine a flashlight into the dark corners of your closet. Back there where you keep the bell-bottoms, ever ready for Woodstock XXX. Further back where your varsity jacket from Ridgemont High has become a feeding station for moths. And up there, behind that box of love letters from the one that got away, where you hide the skin-tight black jeans that you swear you're going to fit into again—some day.

Now cast caution to the wind and pull everything out. We're not saying that you have to throw away the clothes that you haven't worn for the last decade. But there must be a storage place in the basement—or a museum—where you can visit them whenever a wave of nostalgia overcomes you.

"Divide what you've salvaged into fall/winter clothes and spring/summer clothes," says Ken Karpinski of Sterling, Virginia, image consultant to Fortune 500 companies, the U.S. military, and numerous corporate executives, and author of *Red Socks Don't Work*. Subdivide those into piles by apparel. See how closely what you own matches the suggested wardrobe below. Where you find holes in your wardrobe—or actual holes in the garments—

Spring/Summer Wardrobe

Shirts (Short-Sleeve)
Polo shirt
Button-down or straight collar cotton (striped or print)
Linen
Fun and wild print (Hawaiian-style)

Sweaters
Mock turtleneck in high-quality cotton, silk-cotton blend, or silk knit
Cotton crew neck
Boat neck
Sleeveless vest
Cotton sweatshirt

Pants
Linen
Khakis
Shorts (mid-thigh or to knee)
Tropical wool dress trousers

Sport Jackets
Blue blazer
Cotton, linen, or silk (variety of patterns)

Suits
Earth-tone gabardine
Light shade of poplin (cotton-polyester blend, also called wash-and-wear)

Shoes
Casual slip-ons
Boat or deck shoes
Sneakers
Sandals
Cloth or canvas lace-up or slip-on
Buck or suede oxford lace-up

Coats
Denim jacket
Light windbreaker
Washed silk or microfiber, zip-front, golf-style jacket

Accessories
Swimsuits (boxer trunks)
Belts (rope-style)

think about buying items at the start of each season to fill in the gaps.

Peter Walsh, fashion director of *DNR (Daily News Record)*, the newsmagazine of men's retail and fashion, suggests organizing your closet according to the three Ws: work, workout, and weekend. "Think about the various social and business events that you attend," he says, as well as what we used to call play clothes before we grew up and learned to call it sportswear. This will obviously vary depending on your needs. The Wall Street stockbroker will probably own at least half a dozen suits, while the construction worker will own as many sturdy jeans. Let function fill your closet—not whimsy. You'll spend your money more wisely. And you'll probably have room left over to squeeze that varsity jacket back into the back of the closet. But, really, take it from a friend: Lose the bell-bottoms—they have as much chance of making a comeback as Freddie and the Dreamers.

Fall/Winter Wardrobe

Shirts (Long-Sleeve)
Cotton turtleneck

Flannel shirt (plaid or print)

Corduroy shirt (solid or print)

Button-down cotton oxford (solid or striped)

White or blue pinpoint oxford cloth (button-down or spread collar)

Solid or white shirt, cut fuller (variety of weaves and collars)

Denim work shirt (button-down or straight collar)

Three-button polo knit or heavy gauze rugby shirt

Sweaters
(Choose ribbed, cable knit, "fancy pattern," or solid)

V-neck wool

Crew neck

Cardigan

Turtleneck

Pants
Jeans (blue or black)

Khakis (plain front or pleated)

Gray flannel (pleated, cuffed)

Black wool blend or gabardine (pleated, cuffed)

Corduroys (fine, medium, or wide wale)

Plaid or houndstooth

Sport Jackets
Tweed (Harris or houndstooth)

Blue blazer

Camel hair or cashmere (luxury item)

Suits
Pinstripe (worsted)

Blue, brown, tan, or gray worsted

Shoes
Black dress (wing-tip or cap-toe)

Brown semidress suede oxford

Walking
Slip-on (black, brown, or cordovan; penny loafer or tasseled)

Hiking or work boots
Sneakers (depending on your sport: tennis, running, basketball, and so on, or cross-training)

Coats
Waist-length "ski" jacket or parka

Long wool

Raincoat (or trench coat with removable lining)

Accessories
Hats (knit stocking cap or Irish walking hat)

Scarves

Gloves

Earmuffs

Sleeveless down vest

Belts

Hats

A Style Topper

It was President John F. Kennedy who rang the death knell for the modern hat. On a cold January morning in 1961, he broke tradition and chose not to wear a top hat at his inauguration ceremony. Some men's headwear sellers still mourn the day. While President Kennedy may have encouraged many to throw their political hats in the ring, he also encouraged many others to throw their actual hats in the garbage.

President Kennedy did not know what researchers at the U.S. Army later corroborated and mothers everywhere have always told us: Hats keep you warm. The Army study found that you lose from 8 to 50 percent of your body heat through the top of your head, depending on how much energy you're expending.

"It's amazing how smart your mother was," says Murray Hamlet, chief of research support division for the U.S. Army Research Institute of Environmental Medicine in Natick, Massachusetts. "If you want to keep your hands and feet warm, put your hat on."

"And though there is no scientific research on the subject," says Mark Baum, manager of Worth and Worth, the internationally known hat shop in New York City, "more than a few customers have commented that since they have started wearing hats, they have far fewer colds." (For more information and a catalog, call 1-800-HAT-SHOP.)

Men in Hats

The way the winds of style blow today, wearing a hat is strictly optional. No event or situation demands one, outside of being on a baseball team. Which leaves two reasons to wear a hat: to deal with the weather (be it rain, cold, or harsh sun) or to make a fashion statement. In fact, when we asked experts for the perfect closet full of clothes for a man, only one hat was recommended—a knit wool cap for winter.

The sad truth is that most men are not good hat wearers, no matter what the occasion. Maybe it's a dying art that you need to take the initiative to revive. As the English writer Alison Adburgham wrote in *The Bedside Guardian*, "If you are going to wear a hat at all, be decisive, and go the whole hat. In making a courageous choice . . . you have nothing to lose but your head."

All of this isn't to say that hat wearing is moribund; it's a $3-billion-a-year industry in the United States (though we suspect that baseball caps and cowboy hats are fueling much of that). And there are enough hat choices to make your head spin: the porkpie, the Tyrolean, the fisherman's, the straw, the safari, the Panama, the trilby, the fedora, the derby, the bowler, the homburg, the Irish walking, the top, the cowboy, the sombrero, the beret, the coonskin, and the military.

Tips of the Hat

Many of the above hats are strictly for fun, meant for a golf course, fishing stream, or poker game. There's not much guidance we can give you there, except to remind you that

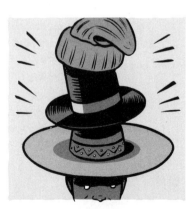

people are actually going to *see* you in them and judge you by them, and that there is a fine line between having a sense of humor and looking plain stupid.

As far as casual winter hats go, again, let your own tastes dictate. However, if you want to keep your ears covered, your choices are limited: a knit cap, a hunter's cap with earflaps, earmuffs, or a coat hood. None scream out "high-class," but all do the job. Our experts' preference: the wool cap, but not so tight as to make you look like a dock worker and not so adorned with college logos and yarn balls on the tip as to make you look like a cheerleader.

Then there are *hats*, those beautiful, satin-lined dress hats that our uncles and grandparents used to wear and that made male movie stars so classy up through the 1950s. These hats are timeless and elegant, and you should consider owning one. "There are three things to keep in mind when deciding on a hat: proportion, fit, and appropriateness," says image consultant Ken Karpinski.

Here are some tricks to pulling off your own hat trick from Peter Annunziata, publisher of *Hat Life Directory* and *Hat Life Newsletter*, the headwear industry's leading publications.

Stand tall—and tapered. A low, tapered crown with a center crease—a homburg, perhaps, or a derby—is what the tall, slender guy needs. A contrasting band around his hat also will help break up the vertical lines of his profile.

Go for a big crown if you're living large. "A tall 200-pounder who stands out in a crowd needs a big hat to balance his figure," Annunziata says. He should wear a fuller crown and a brim that's not too narrow. And he should bend the brim all the way across his face. He'll look good in a semi-homburg or a western-style hat.

Don't sell yourself short. "A short man should always wear a hat," Annunziata says. "He'll always look taller in a hat." A turned-up brim will create the illusion of height, as will a tapered crown. He should avoid turning down the brim so that it covers his eyes, which makes him seem submerged in his hat.

Respect squatter's rights. The wrong hat on a man who's short and squat can be devastating, fashion-wise. A hat can almost literally bury him, or appear that way. He should exercise moderation in all the elements of a hat, from brim to crown to band. If he turns up the brim, it will give him a taller look, adds Annunziata.

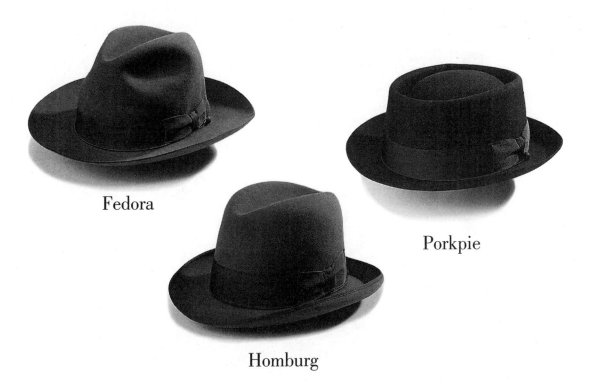

Fedora

Porkpie

Homburg

Capping Things Off

Just when the hat world needed a boost, along came the cap craze. Suddenly, it seemed, every guy in the world was wearing a baseball cap—regardless of whether he played or even liked the sport. Jack Lambert, owner and president of J. J. Hat Center, New York City's oldest hat shop, speculates that the cap became a fashion statement when the first rap groups of the early 1980s started wearing them. Add the push of sports teams to license their logo to hat makers, throw in the popularity of truck drivers' caps, and you have a heady little trend.

"Caps allow you to make a fashion statement fairly inexpensively," says Michele Luna, president of Atlas Headwear in Phoenix, whose family has been making hats for four generations for everyone from the Disney Company to the U.S. Army, with Ralph Lauren, Nike, and Universal Studios in between. "Also, they're a quick way to hide a bad-hair day," she points out.

On the other hand, a comedian once said that a baseball cap immediately knocks 25 points off a man's IQ, and if worn backward, takes off 25 more. As with anything else, be aware of the image you are projecting with a baseball cap.

To get the best deal for the money that you spend on a cap, Luna offers these two suggestions.

Secure the strap. This is the number one problem area. Make sure that the strap is tacked on well. American-made plastic snaps have longer prongs that hold better than the Asian-made ones.

Bend the brim. This is the whole reason to own a cap: We all know that its personality is in how you train the brim to your liking. Fiberboard inner linings are washable, they're flexible, and "they're meant to be played with," Luna says. But the material tends to relax back to its original shape. Once you bend a high-density plastic lining, though, it will stay that way for eternity.

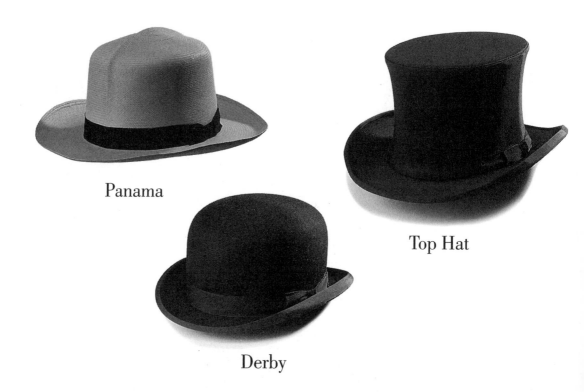

Panama

Derby

Top Hat

Suits

The Rolls-Royce of Style

It may be the most expensive item in your closet. Some of us have only one. We wear it only on very special occasions—regardless of whether it still fits. Others of us wear one to work every day of our lives (hopefully not the same one), like prison uniforms or the steel armor of a knight.

No matter how you feel about them, suits are the Rolls-Royce of your wardrobe, the high-ticket items that are worth every penny that you invest in them.

"The suit remains the uniform of official power," writes art historian Anne Hollander, a fellow of the New York Institute for the Humanities in New York City and author of *Seeing through Clothes* and *Sex and Suits*. "It suggests diplomacy, compromise, civility, and physical self-control. . . . In their pure form they express a confident adult masculinity, unflavored with either violence or passivity."

And, she adds in conversation, they express something else: sex appeal.

"Sexiness doesn't necessarily mean skin-tight and form-fitting," she explains. "The way the suit drapes your body, the suggestive breaks in the lines, the mystery of the wrinkles, the hint of what lies underneath—these are a kind of abstraction of nudity. When worn with confidence and self-assurance, a suit makes a man very appealing."

Suiting Up

These days just buying a suit takes confidence. Consider the choices. Two-piece or three-piece. One-button, two-button, three-button, and even four-button. Wide lapel or narrow

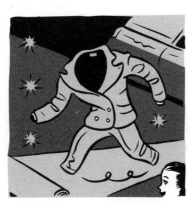

lapel. Single-breasted or double-breasted. And we haven't even touched on pants—or price range. You can spend as little as $130 or as much as $2,000 or more. There *is*, to your relief, an uncomplicated part to all of this. Because suits consist of jackets and pants, much of what you're about to read serves double duty when you go about buying those items of apparel as separates.

The first question clothier Sid Shapiro asks men before he advises them on what type of suit to buy is "What do you do for a living?" This tells you right away that suits are most often associated with work, not play.

Shapiro is president of Syd Jerome, a men's specialty clothier known in Chicago's financial district as the home of the Chicago power suit.

So what's a power suit? More than most of us can afford—but something to aspire to. "It's well-tailored, stylish in a timeless sense," explains Shapiro. "When you walk into a room, people take note of you." It could also have something to do with the price tag: anywhere from $800 to $2,000. Maybe you don't have or want that much power, but the point is to know that a suit can empower you, if you so choose. With that in mind, here are questions that you should ask and the answers that you should hear if you're looking for a good suit.

What type of material is the suit made of? One hundred percent wool is the answer you want to hear if you're looking for quality and comfort, says Mark Alden Lukas, creative director for tailored clothing of Perry Ellis in New York City. However, he adds, small amounts (8 percent) of synthetics blended with wool "can enhance structure and give greater depth and crispness of color."

Is it imported? If so, from where? Most professionals in the menswear business utter the word "Italian-made" with reverence. "Italian tailors are gifted artisans, poets," waxes Murray Pearlstein of Louis, Boston, for

Classic Suits

American ▶

Sometimes called the sack suit, this style is cut straight and full, with lightly padded shoulders (no one will confuse you with an NFL lineman). It has a square front, with the line continuing generally straight through the hips. It has a single shallow center vent in the rear, low-cut armpits, and medium-width lapels. It comes in single-breasted style with two or three buttons in the front. The accompanying pants are without pleats or cuffs. This is as conservative as you can get on a suit.

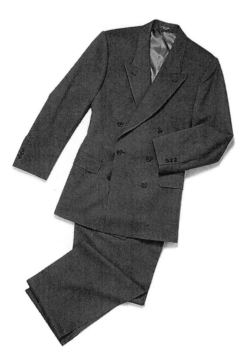

◀ European

Padded shoulders and a snug fit at the waist and hips make this cut look much more provocatively contoured to the V figure of a man. The jacket either has side vents or is non-vented, with high armpits and narrow lapels. The pockets are flapped. It can be either single- or double-breasted. The trousers are pleated with either two or three pleats. Comes in two- and three-button models. This fashion-forward style, as they'd say in Milan, is consistent with the slim and trim look popular in most European clothing. Hefty men should avoid wearing this style.

British or English ▶

This silhouette stays closer to the lines of a man's body. The shoulders are slightly padded, the waist is noticeably nipped in, the back has two deep side vents, and the trousers are usually cuffed and pleated. The pockets are usually angled and flapped. This is a sophisticated but classy look popularized by debonair men like Fred Astaire, Cary Grant, and the Duke of Windsor.

example. Their gift comes from being members of families that have sewn fabrics together for hundreds of years. But, alas, it's a dying art. Today, with globalization of manufacturing procedures, "Made in Italy" could just as likely mean made in Indonesia or Korea or Jersey City. If you want to get really esoteric, though, ask the salesman where the suit was *tailored*. If he says Rome, Milan, or Naples, you can trust that it will fit like a sonnet written only for you.

Is it hand-finished or fused? Fused means that the pieces of the suit fabric are glued together. Hand-finished means they are sewn together by hand. Suits costing less than $500 are usually fused; those above $500 are probably hand-sewn. Ordinarily, hand-finished implies that it's better-made and will last longer—but not always, says Lukas. "Fusing is not necessarily a bad thing, because the quality of fusing has improved," he explains. "Some fusing gives a fabric stability, and sometimes handmade is not perfect."

Still, he suggests that you minimize your gamble by looking for hand-finished suits.

Who is the manufacturer? Among the better American suit makers are Hart Schaffner & Marx and Hickey-Freeman, both part of Hartmarx in Chicago; H. Freeman and Sons of Philadelphia; Hugo Boss, a maker based in Cleveland; and Calvin Klein and Joseph Abboud, both New York City–based.

Is it hand-stitched or machine-stitched? Again, the choice is still the old-fashioned hand stitching. "It has to do with comfort," says Lukas. "The tension of the hand-stitched thread is more forgiving. Machine stitching is rigid." You can tell that the suit is hand-stitched when you see little white stitching on the shoulder.

Look for these signs of poor stitching, whether by hand or machine, says John Larranaga, merchandise development manager for men's clothing and furnishings for

A Vested Interest in Style

In or out of fashion, vests never go out of style, says image consultant G. Bruce Boyer. Worn to match a suit, or in different color or fabric to complement a sport jacket, or simply as an accessory to a white or patterned semidress shirt, here are some basics to wearing a vest that will never go out of style.

- A vest should fit snugly but not so tightly that it constricts your torso. Use that small belt in the back to adjust it to fit comfortably.
- It should cover the waistband of your pants. We shouldn't see your belt or shirt front. It should peak out just above the top of the suit jacket. The points of the shirt collar should not be covered by the vest.
- Leave the bottom button open in deference to King George IV, who forgot to button his before a big shindig and inadvertently instituted a tradition.
- Vests should not be worn unbuttoned under a jacket. After all, what's the point? You lose the whole effect that you're after.

JCPenney: bubbling at the shoulder, collar, or lapels; mismatched patterns; inner linings that are too loose; buttons that are poorly stitched. Dangling thread is *not* a sign of poor stitching—unless you pull it and the garment unravels in your hands.

What are the buttons made of? Plastic or spun polyester buttons are cheap. They crack and break—and always at the most inconvenient moments, or so it seems. Better are horned buttons made from an actual animal's horn, ground to a dust and then mixed with some plastic. Other fine materials are mother-of-pearl and corozzo, a nut material dyed to match the swatch. Image consultant G. Bruce Boyer says that a new ceramic button, developed by none other than Coors Beer and used by Brooks Brothers, is so durable that "you can't break it with a sledgehammer." But we wouldn't recommend that you test it at home.

Sport Jackets

Be a Man of All Seasons

Between the suit and the sweat suit lies the sport jacket. With complementary pants and shirt, with or without a tie, this is the outfit that the vast majority of us wear to work or to social events when we are expected to look like the grown-ups that we're pretending to be.

"A sport jacket gives a man an opportunity to demonstrate he knows how to put an ensemble together," says John Venafro, an assistant technical instructor at Philadelphia College of Textiles and Science and a former menswear buyer and designer. "It's a mature look without being too formal, as in a suit."

The secret of how to look good in a sport jacket is in the fit. "The moment you slip it on, it should feel like a second skin," says Murray Pearlstein of Louis, Boston. "The cut should match the silhouette of your body, close but comfortable."

A tailor's secret that he confides as to how they get that feeling is in the cut of the armholes: They'll make the width wider to compensate for a shorter cut in depth. That way, it fits tightly, but there's room when you lift your arms above your head. This armhole thing is critical because a tailor can't fix it in the fitting room as he can a pant length. What you buy is what you get. Cut too low, the sleeves bind. Cut too narrow, and the upper sleeves pull across the biceps. So consumer be armed.

Abreast of Style

The first question to answer when buying a jacket or a suit is this: Single-breasted or double-breasted? Double-breasted—which means that the

left side of the jacket front overlaps the right side—was a much more popular look prior to World War II. After the war, single-breasted jackets took over because they were less expensive and easier to produce.

Now single and double are both in style, equally appropriate for social events or work, though single-breasted jackets are universally viewed as the traditional look, the standard-bearer of jackets, and double-breasted jackets tend to be saved for dressier occasions. Interestingly, though, the price difference is negligible between single-breasted and double-breasted jackets of the same fabric and quality.

Some men feel that it takes a certain flair to pull off the flashy look of a double-breasted jacket because of the lapels that flare out. But it may have more to do with the buttons. There are usually six buttons, three on each side. On a military uniform, those extra buttons used to mean a higher rank, notes Anne Hollander of the New York Institute for the Humanities. Today, they just mean you like the way they look. Of the three outside buttons, you button either the bottom or middle button.

Another myth is that some men look better in single-breasted rather than double-breasted jackets. Not true anymore, says image consultant Ken Karpinski.

"There used to be a clear line of demarcation," he says. "Shorter and heavier men didn't look good in double-breasted jackets. Now manufacturers have cut the jackets so that they typically button to the lowest button."

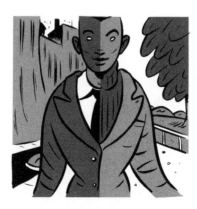

That's called six-to-one. It creates a diagonal line across your body and the illusion of height and trimness. Heavier men who wear single-breasted jackets should always make sure that they can button at least the middle button. "Leave it open and you're showcasing your stomach, which is not what you want to do," Karpinski says.

Lapel widths are about as predictable as the weather in

New England: Wait a minute and they both will change. Whatever we say in *this* moment about whether to go with wide or narrow lapels will change by *this* moment. It's your call. However, when your lapels make you look like a bird about to take flight, you might want to consider toning them down a little.

Venting about Vents

Vents—those slits at the bottom of the back of the jacket—are one of the few details that can distinguish a jacket. As with many other aspects of men's wardrobes, vents were originally designed as part of a military uniform. For soldiers traveling on horseback, the slits in the tails of the military coat let it fall on either side of the saddle, allowing for greater comfort and freedom of motion for the wearer.

Whether you ride a horse or the subway to work, you have a choice of three types of jacket vents: nonvented, single-vented, and double-vented. Here's a look at each.

- *The nonvented jacket.* This creates a streamlined look favored by the

Europeans. The jacket hugs the body, so the body had better be lean and mean or the jacket will pull and have nowhere to go. It's all form and no function. Sit down or try to put your hands in your pant pockets, and the jacket creases and bunches up in the back.

- *The single-vented jacket.* The slit runs up the middle of the jacket back, cuts the wearer down the middle, and creates a boxy sort of look. Slide your hand in a pocket, and the jacket pulls to one side, perhaps revealing things in the rear that you'd rather the rest of the world not view.

- *The double-vented jacket.* A slit on each side of the jacket back adds shape to the garment by emphasizing the outside lines of the body. Those vertical lines make you look taller. With two vents, anyone observing you can see the movement of your legs through the jacket when you walk, creating a sense of fluidity and grace. This is the match of form and function. Given the choice of the three vents,

Single-Breasted Jacket

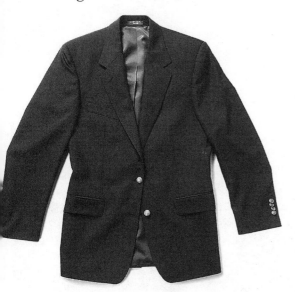

Double-Breasted Jacket

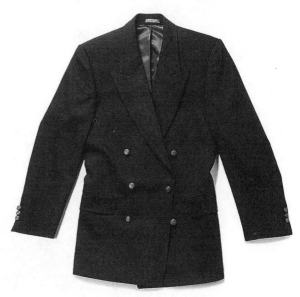

this is the one to pick. One warning, though: This can be a difficult jacket to find. Call a store first to see if they carry this style before making the trip.

Jackets for All Seasons

Since you will probably have more sport jackets than suits, it makes sense to own several varieties, suitable for the four seasons.

Spring/Summer Fabrics

Here's what you need to know to maintain your cool when the weather turns warm.

• *Madras.* A cotton or cotton-silk blend in pastel colors. It runs when washed, so dry-clean only. "Because it wrinkles so easily, this casual jacket is seen as part of the wardrobe of people who can afford to have it pressed a lot," Venafro says. It's worn mostly for casual scenes and goes well with cotton, silk, or linen pants. With light blue or gray pants and a white or light striped shirt, you'll be ready for the polo match, old chap.

• *Linen.* Coarsely woven flax with a nubby, glossy surface. There's no fabric that you will look cooler in—as long as you don't sit, move, or blink an eye. Once you do, the linen will wrinkle—and wrinkle badly—turning you into a disheveled mess. But go ahead—enjoy your minute of casual cool. "For those who are fanatical about looking perfectly pressed, this is *not* the fabric to wear. But for those self-confident enough to know that wrinkled natural fabrics are not a bad character reference, give it a try," says Venafro. The dabbler can meet at the halfway point: Try a blend of linen and silk or wool. This is not a jacket to wear to work; it's perfect, though, for a summer dinner at the shore.

• *Silk.* Lustrous, almost incandescent sheen. "This is a luxurious fabric for holidays and special occasions for evenings and weekends," Venafro says. The type of pants would depend on the grade of silk—the finer the silk, the finer the quality of silk, linen, or wool pants.

• *Seersucker.* Woven, crinkly cotton, most often in blue stripes—if you don't mind

Narrow Lapel	Standard Lapel	Wide Lapel
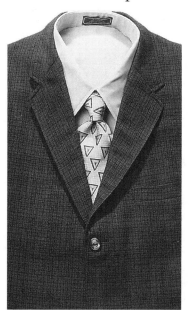	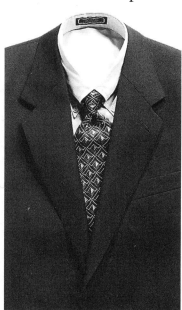	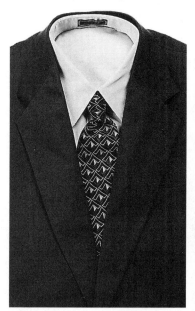

being confused for an escaped con or your Uncle Mortimer from Des Moines. But, suggests Venafro, seersucker makes for a better suit than going solo as a sport jacket.

Fall/Winter Fabrics

When the weather turns cold, here's how to turn up the heat.

• *Serge*. Finely spun worsted wool, usually in dark colors. "There's nothing special about serge," Venafro says. "It's very basic, a safe choice that you can't go wrong with." Which is probably why you see men wearing it everywhere and all the time.

• *Flannel*. Loosely woven luxurious wool that's rich and versatile. This delicate fabric shouldn't be sent to the cleaners too much or it won't last. It's better to brush it out with a brush made for this purpose. "In a bronze brown, black, or navy, this jacket would be great for elegant events just short of formal affairs," Venafro says. With black tie, you can even wear it to black-tie-optional events. Or less formally with piled cotton or corduroy pants and a lamb's wool turtleneck sweater. A finer variety is camel hair, made from the hair of the desert beast interwoven with wool. An even finer flannel is cashmere, the most expensive and the softest of the wool family.

• *Tweed*. Rough and burly wool fabric of several interwoven colors. Weaves are Harris tweed, the coarsest weave, from Scotland's Outer Hebrides Islands; softer Shetland tweed, from the islands of the same name; and Donegal tweed, from Ireland's County Donegal, which has irregular nubs and flecks of color. Patterns include herringbone, the zigzag that resembles a fish's skeleton; houndstooth, a broken but regular check; gun club, large checks woven over smaller ones of a different color; and others. (Tattersall and glen plaid

checks are usually found in suits.) Houndstooth, with its mix of colors, is the most flexible in terms of matching with shirt and pants. It works well with corduroy or bulkier piled cotton pants. As for shirts, "oxford stripes are fine, but stay subtle with patterns," advises Venafro. Large checked shirts would work because they don't compete with the small patterns that the interwoven fabrics make.

• *Corduroy*. Cotton ribbed in various widths known as wales. Venafro says the same of corduroy sport jackets that he does for seersucker: better as a suit—"unless you go very, very casual, like with jeans and turtlenecks."

What in Blazers Is Going On?

According to one well-worn legend, the blazer was named when a British captain of a nineteenth-century naval vessel, the H.M.S. Blazer, ordered his sloppily dressed crew to shape up or ship out—and forced them to wear blue serge jackets with gold metal buttons.

Apocryphal or not, it is true that the uniform look of blazers makes them both easy and hard to wear.

"The thing that is going to make one blazer stand out over another is good tailoring—an excellent fabric and a wonderful cut," says Murray Pearlstein of Louis, Boston.

The most common fabric is serge, a weave of wool. It's comfortable and lightweight and has a dull luster that many men like. Expect to pay between $125 and $140.

If you want to borrow against your retirement fund to finance an elegant blazer that will last the rest of your life, Pearlstein recommends a flannel or cashmere fabric. "It has a soft nap that makes you look relaxed, like you're in charge of the blazer—not vice versa," he says. "It's a little weightier than serge but, wow, what a feel." And how's this price tag for a wow: $800 and up.

Pants

Stepping Out in Style

If there is one article of clothing that defines a man, it is his pants. They are the universal symbol of masculinity. After all, how would we know which door to enter if not for the pants worn by the little silhouette on entrances to public bathrooms?

Pants are confidence and self-assurance. When we ask who wears the pants in the family, we're not really curious about who has zipped up this morning. We're inquiring about who makes the decisions, who has the power.

But our pants do a lot more than work overtime as metaphors for masculinity. They are the workhorses of our wardrobe, probably taking more of a beating than any other clothes we wear. Since we were kids, we've left grass stains on the knees, torn the pockets, frayed the bottoms. When we got older, we were no kinder, leaving permanent wallet scars, abusing pockets that double for desk drawers, working that zipper to death to pass about two quarts of urine every day.

Sales of men's pants reflect the pivotal role that they play in our wardrobes. In the first half of 1996, for example, pants were one of the fastest-growing segments in the retail apparel market, according to NPD Consumer Purchase Panel.

It's probably because of all this that fit and durability have often been higher in men's minds than style. But there's no reason why you can't have both.

Getting Fit

Whether you call them pants, trousers, or slacks (*that* depends on your generation),

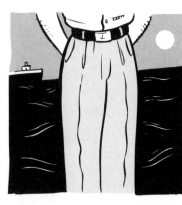

whether you're talking about knockabout Dockers or the finest dress pants made, fit begins at the top—at the waist.

Short and simple, trousers should be worn on the waist, not below, on the hip. Jeans are the lone exception to the rule. Anything else and you're actually doing yourself a disservice, warns menswear designer Alan Flusser. "Every man, no matter how thin, has a slight bulge in his stomach," he explains. "When trousers are worn on the waist, they pass smoothly over this bulge in an even drape," emphasizing your thinness. Men only accentuate their gut when they wear pants below their waists. If you have trouble keeping your pants up that high, fasten the button inside your pants that crosses your zipper. That's what it's designed for: to act as a kind of secret suspender.

Get the wrong fit, and you could suffer more than pained glances. You could suffer from "tight pants syndrome," a malady observed by Octavio Bessa, M.D., assistant professor of medicine at New York Medical College in Valhalla, New York. This was especially true with patients who reported bloating, heartburn, and other abdominal discomfort for whom he could find no other cause. The syndrome was most prevalent among men whose waists were two inches or more larger than the waists of the pants that they wore. He recommends a quick way to test yourself for tight pants syndrome: Buy a pair of pants one size larger than you normally wear. If the symptoms go away, the problem was in your pants. If the trousers don't easily reach your waist, it may be due to a short "rise"—the distance between the base of your crotch and the waistband. Ask for trousers with a higher rise, suggests image consultant G. Bruce Boyer. If it appears that you could fit King Kong's "family jewels" in that space along with your own, the rise is too long.

The Belt Way

Accessories are the fun part. And belts are no exception.

"The right belt can tie your whole outfit together," says Mark Alden Lukas of Perry Ellis. "It's the kind of accessory that can be as bland as salt, or it can spice up your whole wardrobe like an exotic herb."

Like a good seasoning, it should harmonize and blend, but when examined closely, it should make a strong statement on its own. Here's a quick tip: The color of the belt should match the color of your shoes.

Unless you're morally opposed to wearing animal skin, optimally you want genuine leather, says Scott Weiner, a member of the Belt Association and vice-president of Tiger Accessories, a manufacturer in Bay Shore, New York, which makes boys' and men's belts for chain stores such as Kmart and JCPenney and licensed brands such as Beverly Hills Polo Club. He says that you can trust that stamp on the back of the belt; the Federal Trade Commission strictly regulates what it stamps as leather and its grading.

Full-grain is top-of-the-line. It usually comes from the stiff shoulder or softer side of the cow. Split cowhide is at the low end. Alligator, crocodile, lizard, and snakeskins—the exotics, as they're called in the industry—are at the even higher end.

About a third of the belts sold in the United States are priced between $20 and $35. Another third are from $35 to $50. The last third are divided between expensive (over $50) and inexpensive (below $20). To get the look of a $75 belt for the price of a $20 belt, Weiner says, some chain stores will treat a lower-grade leather—it's called tanning—to give it that extra grainy look and feel.

Here are some other suggestions when you want your belt to do more than hold up your pants.

Beware big buckles. They draw attention to an area of your body that you might not necessarily want people staring at, namely, that extra 10 pounds in your gut. Anyway, the brass replica of the Inca Sun God with a turquoise third eye that you brought back from Sedona, Arizona, won't work with your pinstripe suit, no matter how committed you are to economic growth in America's Sunbelt region.

Get the right size. A belt should be long enough, when buckled, to reach the first loop but not the second, says menswear designer Alan Flusser. Dress belts should be between 1¼ and 1½ inches in width.

Color-coordinate. Aside from matching your shoes, the color of your belt should be darker than the clothes you're wearing. Light-colored belts connote sportier, more casual attire, as do rougher grained and textured leather. Buckles should be brass or silver.

Skin it. If you go for leather or reptile skin, look for a belt that has no body scars, blemishes, burns, scratches, or other imperfections. Those will cost more but last longer.

Then there's the question of dress. Relax, it has nothing to do with skirts. "*Dress* refers to the side on which a man places his more intimate anatomic parts," explains Boyer. "You either dress left or dress right (for inexplicable reasons, most men dress left). That's why there's a tad more room on the left leg of the trouser." If you find that you need more room there, confide in your trusty tailor.

Since the crotch area gets so much usage—with all that shifting from dress right to dress left, sitting and standing and the friction of the material when you walk—good pants add a piece of fabric to the inner lining from the crotch down. It's called—no need to mince words here—a crotch piece. "Pants with a crotch piece are a true hallmark of quality," says Mark Alden Lukas of Perry Ellis. "It reduces abrasion and prolongs the life of the pants."

The next area critical to a good fit is your seat. If your waist is proportionately bigger than your rear end, there will be enough room in the seat of your pants to hide a sack of potatoes back there. If your rear end is proportionately bigger than your waist, your pants will be too tight. The solution, if you just can't find pants in

a department store that fit right, is to hire a tailor to smooth the seat so that it's comfortable when you're sitting or standing. But remember—in

Khakis: Timeless Classics

Some men seem to live in khakis. And who can blame them? Those light brown pants work. They work hard. And they work with everything—with blue blazer or tweed sport jacket and tie. With all variety of shirts: short-sleeve polo, denim work, button-down oxford, T-shirt, or sweatshirt. With sweaters and turtlenecks. With every pattern: stripes, solids, checks, plaids. Cheap, easy to wash and dry, no need to iron: the perfect pants. And available in any color you want—as long as it's . . . khaki.

"They're the ultimate casual alternative to jeans," says Mark Alden Lukas of Perry Ellis. "Slightly dressier but not a dress trouser. The color is a classic neutral. It goes with so much. And the fabric is so durable."

Khakis have been through the wars—literally. Army-issued khakis (once called chinos because the cotton drill cloth that they were made of came from China) first appeared on college campuses back in the late 1940s and

Pleats

Plain-Front

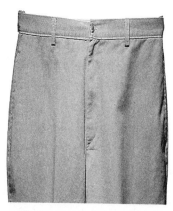

Double-Forward Pleat

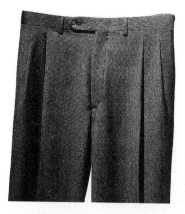

early 1950s, worn by GIs returning from World War II. But they had been part of military uniforms 100 years earlier.

In 1846 Sir Harry Lumsden of the British Army, in command in India, realized that the sparkling white cotton drill uniforms that his troops wore made them sitting ducks for snipers, according to image consultant G. Bruce Boyer. He also caught on that those men who ignored Army policy and let their clothes get dirty blended better with the dusty terrain and ended up living longer. So Lumsden broke rank and ordered his troops to dye their uniforms—some say with tea, others with river mud. The resulting color was the perfect camouflage. Its name comes from the Persian word for dirt or dust—*khak*.

By 1884 the khaki color was patented. The British War Office officially adopted the material for troops in active service. The American Army followed suit, making it general issue in 1914 just in time for World War I.

chalking in the cut lines.

The leg should be long enough to reach the top of your shoe, just enough to break the crease of the pant. It should break over the instep of the shoe in front and drop to within an inch of the top of the heel in the back.

While suggested pant widths ebb and flow according to fashion trends, the changes only measure in quarter- and half-inches—not enough to throw out all your old pants, Boyer says. Unless you've kept those bell-bottoms from your love-in days. "The trouser leg should fall straight and generally follow the natural contour of your body," he notes. "If you have a 30- to 34-inch waist, your pants should be about 19 inches at the knee and 17½ inches at the bottom."

Here are several surefire ways to tell if you're still floundering over the concept of fit.

• The front pockets, whether on the seam, diagonal, or horizontal, will bow out from the pants. They are screaming, "You're stretching our capacity. Go either to the next size up or the gym."

• You won't be able to cram a finger between your waistband and your waist. It's one

case your tailor doesn't—taking in or letting out your seat will alter the fit of the legs and crotch, so make sure that he aligns everything before

Triple-Forward Pleat

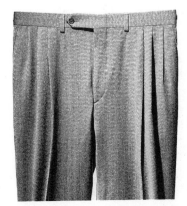

Double-Reverse Pleat

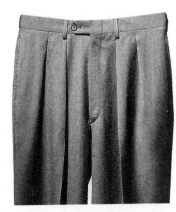

Box Pleat

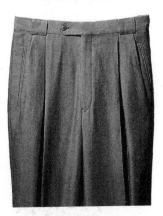

thing when this test fails with your old high school marching band uniform. It's quite another when your finger gets stuck in the Dockers that you fought your way into this morning.

- If people behind you start giggling when you bend over, you may be exposing more of yourself than you—and certainly they—would care to see. Odds are that your pants are riding too low, probably because you're not wearing them around your waist, probably because they won't fit around your waist, probably because you bought them in a size too small for your waist.

- If the pleats of your pants open too much, there probably is not enough material to accommodate your girth.

- If people comment on your mismatched socks while you're still standing, your pants are too short. If folks ask if you're standing in a hole, your pants are too long and you can finally whine that oldest of tailor's sayings, "Sam, you make the pants too long."

The Grand Design

There's far more to pant design, of course, than just the long and short of it. Here are three other key considerations.

1. Pleats. Pants come in two varieties: plain-front and pleated. "Properly fitting plain-front pants can make you look slimmer if the pockets are on-seam," Lukas says.

But pleated pants "have long been the choice of well-dressed men," says Flusser. And they have become the most popular style in pants, whether casual or dress. The utilitarian and aesthetic arguments for pleats far outweigh those for the plain-front.

For starters, pleats allow more fullness and room through the thighs, knees, and bottom. When you sit down, they expand like an accordion to make room for your expanding hips. They reduce wrinkling in your lap—good news if you drive to work or you sit all day. They allow a graceful draping of the cloth, and

their vertical lines create an illusion of thinness.

You've probably been too busy worrying about the national debt to realize that pants usually come with two or three pleats on each side of the zipper, each affording increasingly more room. ("The mature man with a full physique should avoid triple pleats, for they draw way too much attention to his mid-section," advises Lukas.) There are forward (sometimes called English) pleats, which open toward the zipper, and reverse pleats, which open toward the pockets. Lukas theorizes that reverse pleats "create a cleaner look." Another variation is box pleats, which resemble squares.

2. Cuffs. And now the question that has perplexed man since the beginning of tailored time: Cuffs or no cuffs? Our experts recommend cuffs. One good reason is that they add weight to the bottom of your pants, helping to keep the crease lines running straight down. To elongate the look of your legs, go cuffless. To shorten the look, get cuffed, suggests image consultant Ken Karpinski. In the end, as with much of style, it comes down to personal preference. If you prefer going through life off the cuff, do it with gusto.

Once you decide on cuffs, you're ready for the deeper philosophical question: How wide? Flusser suggests that men 5 feet 10 inches or under should wear cuffs 1⅝ inches wide; taller men should wear cuffs 1¾ inches wide. And you thought that football was a game of inches; style is a game of eighth-inches.

3. Pockets. For comfort, accessibility, and utility, men's favorite pocket angles away from the seam about an inch or so. "It's easy to get into and out of," says Lukas. "It tilts at the same angle as the hand." Fashion designers prefer the on-seam pocket, since its lines are the cleanest. But, frankly, it's harder to get into and out of. So let *them* wear that style. True-grit men wear the western-style pocket, which cuts horizontally across the front. That may be fine for cowboys who never get phone messages and have nowhere to make change. Besides, it's not like you need a key to start your horse. But it's highly impractical for the rest of us.

Jeans

Wearing an American Original

In the American Wing of the Metropolitan Museum of Art in New York City, you'll find precious paintings, sculptures, furniture, and other artifacts that offer fascinating insights into the history of the United States.

But if you truly want to understand the twentieth century, look in your clothes closet, suggests Richard Martin, curator of the museum's Costume Institute. It's likely that you'll find the most enduring symbol hanging there, perhaps a bit faded and blue.

"Jeans are the consummate American icon," Martin says. "They are symbolic of the lifestyle of the twentieth century. Created for the rigor and exactitude of work, they command our imagination of the relaxed, casual, and leisured. No flag, no costume, no pageant has ever more embodied a nation and its ambition and social idealism."

The Making of a Myth

Those blue denims are—quite literally—woven into the fabric of American life, an indispensable part of any man's wardrobe. According to a survey of 300 men and 100 women, commissioned by VF Corporation, which owns Lee, Wrangler, and Riders jeanswear brands, one-third of those polled said that they owned 10 or more pairs of jeans.

Why are the faded blues so popular? Steve Goldstein, vice-president of marketing and research for San Francisco–based Levi Strauss and Company, takes a cultural stab at that question: "The fundamental characteristic of jeans is that at their heart they allow you to be who you are.

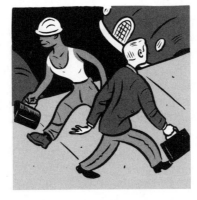

Nothing's more appealing to a guy than that. They mold to you. You can write your own story in them."

Plus they're comfortable, durable, and versatile—you can wear them with a silk shirt or a sweatshirt—and they tell a story of their own that appeals to every self-made man's frontier spirit.

It's the story of a Bavarian immigrant who arrived in San Francisco in 1853 during the Gold Rush and figured out that there was gold in them thar pants that held up to the hard life of a miner. So the fellow, one Levi Strauss, turned tough tenting canvas into waist-high overalls. The trousers were soon being made in a durable cotton, woven in Nimes in Southern France. The material was called *serges de Nimes*, which became the colloquial *denim* (*serges* is French for any fabric with a diagonal weave). The word *jeans* is thought to be a bastardization of *Genoese*, in reference to the Italian sailors whose uniforms included blue denims. When a Nevada tailor suggested that Strauss use a rustproof copper rivet to secure the frequently torn pocket seams, all the elements were in place.

Finding the Right Size

Now, along with Levi's and the VF brands, you have Brittania, Bugle Boy, Cherokee, Esprit, Guess?, H.I.S., Sasson, Sergio, Tommy Hilfiger, and others all scrambling to get you into their pants, so to speak.

In the new generation of jeans, you don't have to drag your brand new stiff-as-a-rail dark blues around the barn floor a couple hundred times to give them that much-desired lived-in faded look. Many companies now use enzymes to soften and fade the fabric, giving them a stone-washed look. There's also sand-blasting, yet another way to make new look old. Another innovation is called mill-washing, which allows manufacturers to remove the starch in the fabric without removing the dark blue dye. So you can look like you've been riding the range all day without feeling that way.

It's stunning to see how prices can vary between all the different jeans brands. Primarily, more money buys you a more prestigious label—and not much else. Yes, a better pair of jeans has minor embellishments like additional seaming, extra pockets, more studs, better softening processes, a slightly different design. Basically, though, denim is denim; there just aren't that many grades of quality.

With so many choices, men have trouble deciding which jeans to buy. The VF survey found that, when shopping for jeans, a third of the men polled tried on up to 10 pairs at a time, and 5 percent confessed to bringing as many as 20 pairs into the fitting room.

The problem with finding the right fit is that while all men may be created equal, not all 34/32 jeans are. "As with any handmade product, there will be variances in waist and seam," explains Goldstein. "No two jeans are exactly alike."

"Stick with reputable brands that specialize in jeans," suggests Dr. Susan Ashdown of Cornell University. Her reasoning is that those companies do extensive research testing how the denim fabric behaves when washed. The shrinkage will be in the length or inseam, which also effects the crotch but not the waist. Go for a pair that's about two inches larger than you need in the waist and leg, suggests Norman Karr, executive director of Jeanswear Communications, a New York City–based information clearinghouse representing major denim producers and jeans manufacturers.

Other than that, adds Dr. Ashdown, you just have to try them on. Even if you've bought

Getting in Shape

Jeanswear makers and marketeers have a field day creating terminology to let us know that we can still fit into our jeans at any age. Here's a translation.

• *Traditional or regular fit.* This is the classic, cut to the contour of your body. God willing, your body makes the cut. This straight-leg version usually runs about 16 inches wide at the ankles. Great for young men whose percentage of body fat runs in the single digits.

• *Relaxed or easy fit.* Generally gives you about a half-inch more room in the seat, thigh, leg, and knee, with a slight taper to 15 inches at the ankle. Perfect for men in their thirties and forties who don't yet look like they've swallowed a bowling ball but aren't exactly svelte either.

• *Loose or baggy fit or wide-leg.* Room for you and a friend, with as much as four extra inches at the seat and thigh. In loose fits, the ankle tapers; wide legs are nicknamed pipes because the legs are that wide. This look is for either very young hip-hoppers hiding stolen merchandise or very old hippies hiding their gut.

One other point of confusion is the cut of the jeans' lower leg. Here are some definitions.

• *Straight cut.* Means that the pant leg has the same width all the way down the seam, generally cut pretty tight, and recommended only for slim guys.

• *Flair.* Adds about an inch in pant-leg width beginning just below the knee. This provides a slight flair, as opposed to a bell-bottom, which has several inches of flair. Still, the flair cut has generally had its day and is not worn that much at all anymore.

• *Boot cut.* Also called the cowboy cut (for example, Wrangler's Cowboy Cut "original"), is cut a little wider at the ankle to accommodate high boots that you'll be line dancing in.

the same size before, each pair will fit differently. As for the critical fit around your hopefully sexy derriere, she suggests using fitting rooms with three-way mirrors: "That's the only way that you'll see your behind the way that other people see it."

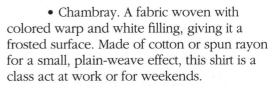

Shirts

Keep Something Stylish up Your Sleeve

We take quite seriously giving someone the shirt off our back. As though relinquishing that item of apparel was as selfless an act as giving your own flesh.

"Your shirt defines who you are more than any other item," says Mark Weber, vice-chairman of Phillips–Van Heusen Corporation in New York City, the country's largest shirt maker, and author of *Dress Casually for Success . . . for Men.* "You may not wear a jacket or tie all the time, but—at least in public—you're going to be wearing a shirt."

To be fair, "shirt" may cover your back, but the term barely covers the subject. You could be talking about any of the following:

• Gingham. A plain-weave fabric of cotton in checks, plaids, or stripes. The fabric serves well for a multitude of purposes, from work to weekend to just kicking around the house.

• White dress. In its many subtle shades, fabrics, and collar styles, the white dress shirt is always right, never wrong, at work or for important social occasions. In a pinch, you can wear it with a sweater and khakis and fit right in, too.

• Silk. Slinky product of the industrious silkworm. Resilient and wrinkle-resistant (but not wrinkle-free—try wearing it on a hot day and peeling it off your back), this has become synonymous with a rich Hollywood look, especially when buttoned at the neck, sans tie. Wear it for that upscale casual event, like meeting Cindy Crawford for a drink.

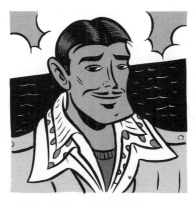

• Chambray. A fabric woven with colored warp and white filling, giving it a frosted surface. Made of cotton or spun rayon for a small, plain-weave effect, this shirt is a class act at work or for weekends.

• Oxford. A modified plain- or basket-weave cotton fabric that originated in Oxford, England. This is the ground zero of shirts, everyone's point of reference, whether with a suit and tie for corporate takeovers or with a crew neck sweater for homecoming reunions.

• Flannel. A loosely woven fabric with a napped surface that hides the weave, made primarily of wool or cotton. This casual shirt says outdoorsy woodsman, even if the closest you get to the woods is watching reruns of *The Life and Times of Grizzly Adams*.

• Corduroy. A plain- or twill-weave fabric of polyester, cotton, rayon, or blends with a cut-pile surface of wide and narrow wales. Like its cousin flannel, this warmest of cotton materials is a logical, cold-weather, casual option. Known as the velvet of the poor, its name derives from the French *cour du roi*, or "court of the kings," and was woven in the hunting outfits of servants.

• Denim. A twill-weave fabric in cotton or a blend of fibers. Extremely sturdy, this fabric was first produced in eighteenth-century Nimes, France—which means that it came *de Nimes*, hence its Americanized name. With a tie, tweed sport jacket, and khakis, you'll fit into any Casual Friday in any office on the planet.

• Polo. A pullover with two or three buttons extending from an attached collar. It was first worn by polo players in the early twentieth century. Now the brand name, Polo, has become a household word. And it's the best-selling shirt in most shirt departments. Wear it for tennis or any other sport, under an informal sport jacket, or with almost any pair of casual pants you own, from jeans to wool dress pants. Its close cousin is the rugby shirt, great for those touch football games.

• Hawaiian. The classic would be a 1940s rayon gabardine, with a print of big flowers in full color in full blossom, with a parrot in there somewhere. You can pay big bucks for the originals, if you can find them in secondhand shops in Maui or on Madison Avenue. Imitations can be fun for sheer effect when you want to draw attention to yourself. When folks laugh when they see you, remember that they're laughing with you, not at you.

• T-shirt. This ubiquitous staple—short-sleeved (or sleeveless for real hunks), collarless, cotton affairs—started as undershirts but soon came out from undercover when some marketing genius realized that if you stenciled your company's name or logo on the chest, you could trick men into being walking free ads. And we took the bait.

Collaring a Great Shirt

To find out what makes a shirt look great on you, start at the top. You wouldn't be sticking your neck out if you concluded that the key is the collar.

"The collar frames a man's face," says Murray Pearlstein of Louis, Boston. "It's so pivotal to the visual impression you make because people look at your face first, your clothes second."

The general rule of thumb is not to wear collars that are shaped the same as your face. So a roundish face should not wear round collars; you'll only accentuate the same shape.

Like women who wear uncomfortable bras, many men assume that tight collars come with the territory of being a guy. In a study a few years back, Susan M. Watkins, professor in the textiles and apparel department of Cornell University in Ithaca, New York, found that 67 percent of men working in law offices and business firms wore neckwear that was too tight.

It doesn't have to be that way, says Mor-

timer Levitt of the Custom Shop, if men would, first, admit that when they gain weight they'll probably need a larger neck size and, second, realize that the neck size on the label when they buy it is lying. Shirt manufacturers allow for about 2.5 percent total shrinkage from washing. "That means that a 15½ collar actually measures almost 16 inches when you get it and shrinks to 15½," he says. So if it fits just right when you buy it, it will be just wrong after repeated washing.

Not only will the wrong size collar make you look bad but also it will make you see badly. Tight neckwear can decrease a man's visual performance, according to Watkins's study. She also found that visibility does not return to normal immediately after the neckwear is removed. The explanation is that the shirt and tie press against the carotid arteries of the neck, blocking blood flow to the brain.

Shop Smart, Look Sharp

Once you've made the right collar, you're ready to learn about the finer points of shirts.

Plead for more pleats. Weber can name a number of specifics to look for—buttons on sleeve plackets (the slits near the cuffs), locker loops on the shirt back, extra replacement buttons at the bottom of the shirt—but "the single most important" detail is pleats in the cuff and in the back. "Pleats afford movement and, therefore, comfort," he explains. "They also require extra fabric, so they cost more." Look for box pleats, which descend from the middle of the back of the shirt, not tuck pleats (folds near the shoulders), which are more for effect than movement.

Look for proportion. Less-expensive shirts look square when you hold them up, says Christine Walter, men's sportswear buyer for Nordstrom in King of Prussia, Pennsylvania. "They look out of proportion." A shirt shouldn't be as wide as it is long—unless that's what your body looks like. There should be length in the shirttails, especially since it will shrink, Walter says.

Check the armpit. This is an area that gets a lot of wear and tear. It's logical that it wears out first. "Look under the arm for tight stitching," suggests Walter.

Try the 5 percent solution. Okay, so we have established beyond reasonable doubt that 100 percent cotton is the fabric of choice. Cotton shirts look and feel terrific, and they absorb sweat. And the sales figures back it up: In 1995, 61 percent of the men's dress shirts sold were made of cotton, according to research that the NPG Group conducted for Cotton. But don't reject shirts that are made with some synthetics, encourages Walter. "Nowadays new synthetics are becoming more sophisticated," she says. "Five percent rayon, silk, or polyester will cut down wrinkling, increase durability, and won't take away from the look of a shirt."

Look for "top-fused" collars. This is a technique for connecting the collar to the rest of the shirt that "practically guarantees a wrinkle-free collar for the life of the shirt," Weber says. Here's how to tell if the collar is top-fused: Lift up the collar. Try to separate the front from the back of the collar. If you can't, it's top-fused. "It will maintain a stiff look but a soft feel," adds Weber.

Hit the links. "There is nothing more elegant than French cuffs," says Weber. If you want to project a persona that says dapper in-the-know power broker, this detail will do it. Now for the detail of the detail: the cuff links. The secret to stylish cuff links is to "keep it simple," says image consultant G. Bruce Boyer. "You just want to

White Knight of the Night

If the collar is the frame, a white shirt is the tabula rasa. "It's the blank canvas on which your face is painted," says Mark Weber of Phillips–Van Heusen Corporation. "White is the most flattering color for any man."

Here's a quick rundown of the fabrics that can turn your white shirt into a Picasso.

Broadcloth. The fibers of this cotton fabric are woven tightly, giving it a soft finish and lots of versatility. Example: Perry Ellis spread-collar broadcloth.

Oxford. This cotton weave is a bit rougher to the touch, making it better for less-formal situations, like Casual Friday. The texture works well with wool and woven ties, and jackets with texture like tweeds. Example: Kenneth Gordon pinpoint oxford.

Linen. Yes, it wrinkles. But yes, it also is a wonderful fabric against your skin in the warmer months. One caution: A bulky tie will overpower the collar. Example: AKA Eddie Bauer 100 percent linen.

Cotton/poly blend. Using only 5 percent polyester doesn't mean that you've sold out to the multinationals. What you lose in breathability you gain in a wrinkle-free environment—at least in your shirt. Example: Arrow cotton/poly blend.

White dress shirts range from $15 to $100 and more. "The more you pay, the more you should expect in the quality of the fabric and the quality of workmanship," says image consultant Ken Karpinski. Unless it's really great fabric, Karpinski adds, if you're paying more than $50, you're probably paying for the designer's label.

see a flash of silver or gold." Get cuffs that have both matching front and back, not the clip-on style.

Choosing the Right Collar

The Button-Down ▶

The collar points button to the shirt. This collar has come to represent a state of mind as much as a style. "Button-down" means conservative, straight-ahead, play by the rules. It's the Ivy League look. "One of its problems is that the collar buckles as the day wears on and gives a somewhat sloppy appearance," says Mark Weber of Phillips–Van Heusen Corporation. It looks best with jackets with natural or "unconstructed" shoulders and with a tie featuring a bigger Windsor knot. It works well with most face shapes. But keep in mind that the longer the points of the collar, the more round the face should be. Long faces should wear shorter points.

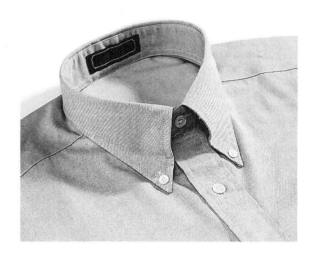

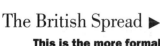

◀ The Spread

It has a wider gap between the points and is more rigid than the straight collar. "This collar should always be worn with a tie," suggests Weber. Remember this: The wider the spread of the collar, the more formal the occasion it should be worn for. This is a good choice for men with thin faces. Because of the spread, tie a half or full Windsor knot with this collar.

The British Spread ▶

This is the more formal cousin of the spread collar. The distance between points is significantly wider than the standard spread. That makes it a smart choice for guys with thin faces, but it's not flattering to men with round faces. Like the standard spread, this one should always be worn with a tie. Because of the extra room for a knot, go with a full Windsor.

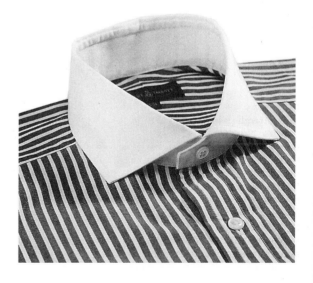

The Tab ▶

This collar is more appropriate for formal and traditional occasions because of the rigid look it creates, propping the tie up and holding it stiffly in place. Men with short, thick necks shouldn't wear tab collars. You can get the same effect by wearing a collar pin under your tie. The knot should be a four-in-hand; nothing else will fit correctly. For best effect, wear a tab collar if you have a medium- to long-shape face.

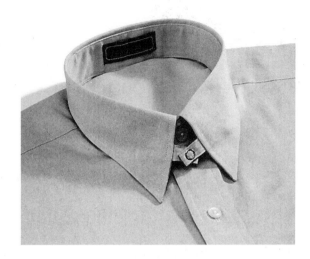

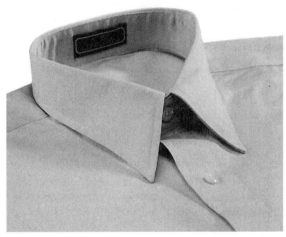

◀ The Straight or Point

The most common type, this long collar has the most variations of length. "Wear it any- where, anytime," says Weber. "It's dressy but not necessarily formal." Pressed with a light starch, this collar will hold up all day. Men with round faces should wear a medium- to long- point, narrow-spread collar. Those with square faces should wear a deeper, rounded collar, or a narrow-spread collar with long points. Good news for all guys: This collar fits all face shapes, and it works well with any tie knot.

The Banded ▶

Proving that you should never throw away old styles—even 100-year-old styles—this was how all shirts looked in the days of detachable collars. Now (without the attached collar), it's considered a chic alternative in dressy and formal settings. It looks great on casual flannel shirts as well. Long-necked men should wear higher-banded collars; short-necked men should wear lower-banded collars. And here's more good news: no tie required. In fact, ties are strictly forbidden. One caution: This collar is not for men with round faces. The lack of vertical lines makes it less than flattering on them.

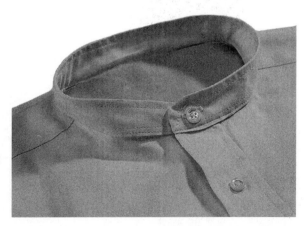

Ties

It's Knot Hard to Express Yourself

The ever-flamboyant nineteenth-century Irish playwright Oscar Wilde best summed up what every man intuitively knows about ties. "A well-tied tie is the first serious step in life," he said.

Another grand dandy, George Bryan "Beau" Brummell, took the step so seriously that it's said that he sometimes knotted dozens of ties, undoing the failures, dropping them at his feet until he had in one single movement crafted an absolutely perfect work of art.

Maybe you're not that obsessive about your tie. At least we hope not. But chances are that you could stand to pay a little more attention to what you wear around your neck.

"Ties are the sole touch of sartorial fantasy allowed in the masculine wardrobe, and they constitute a veritable stylistic language for users of all ages and backgrounds," French fashion writer François Chaille states in *The Book of Ties*.

That may explain why some 95 million ties are sold in the United States annually, generating more than $800 million in retail sales. It may also explain why so many celebrities—dead and alive—are tied into the tie thing: Jerry Garcia, Miles Davis, Rush Limbaugh, Frank Sinatra, and John Lennon have all lent their names to lines of ties.

Pick the Right One

There also appears to be utility in ties. "Ties are the best way for a man to make that blue shirt look different than the last time he wore it," says Jerry Andersen, executive director of the Neckwear Association of

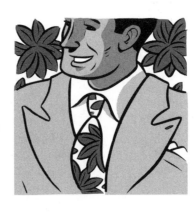

America. "And they're a great way to advertise your personality—conservative, flashy, casual, formal." Yet many of us get choked up when it comes to picking the tie that expresses us best.

"I see it every day of my life: Men have no concept of how to pick ties," says image consultant Ken Karpinski. "They see a sea of 5,000 ties in a department store and are nearly paralyzed by indecision." If rigor mortis sets in when you're picking a tie, Karpinski suggests these steps.

Strike a match. Identify colors in the shirt or jacket that you plan to wear and find matches in the ties that you're interested in. This may be harder than you think, especially for the 6 percent of men who are color-blind.

Be an isolationist. A tie can't be all things to all colors. Choose the one color in a shirt or jacket that you want to accentuate and match that color to the tie.

Turn up the volume. Find the tie that has the most amount of the color that you want to accentuate.

Get coordinated. Make sure that the pattern of the tie is compatible with the shirt or jacket. Avoid what's called tracking. That's when the stripes in the tie are the same width as the jacket or shirt but go at right angles to each other, appearing to form a crisscross pattern.

In the Know

So, really, what *is* the difference between a $10 tie and a $50 tie? Plenty, says Andersen.

"But it's not as easy as you think to discern those differences," he says. The more expensive the tie, he explains, the more it should have of the following qualities: a "substantially beefy hand" (meaning a heavier material); elasticity when you tug it; a full lining, rather than just a thin strip; a fine "registration" of the print (in other words, those parrots or protozoa shouldn't be blurry); hand stitching as

Bow Ties: For the Man with True Character

Think about great men in bow ties: Harvard economist John Kenneth Galbraith, former U.S. Senator Paul Simon, media mogul Chris Whittle, Superman sidekick Jimmy Olsen, comic strip character Archie. These are unique men who stand apart. "A bow tie is very idiosyncratic," says image consultant Ken Karpinski. "People in professions where individuality is prized wear them."

If that's the statement that you want to make—a true character with character—go ahead and wear a bow tie any old time you want, Karpinski suggests. Just make sure that you have the creative goods to back it up. Otherwise, he adds, "you'll come off as a buffoon."

If you pass the character test, there are two things to bear in mind, says menswear designer Alan Flusser. The bow tie's width should not extend beyond the outer edge of your eyes or the breadth of your collar, whichever is wider. Second, tie the tie yourself rather than wearing a pre-tied tie. Wearing one of those clip-ons "is like letting someone else forge your signature," he adds. Of course, then you have to learn how to tie the bow. But that's not as hard as you think. Just follow these easy instructions.

With the tie around your neck and the ends hanging down, place the right end over the left end, leaving the right end slightly longer.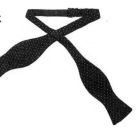

Take the right end and bring it up under the left end so that it is facing straight up.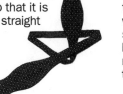

While the right end remains straight up, fold the left end up with the outside showing and bring it over the right end toward the left side.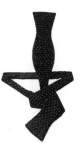

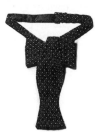 With the left end folded up into a bow on the left side, bring the right end over the left end so it is now pointing down toward the floor. The left end should be parallel to the floor.

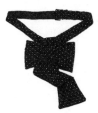 Bring the right end, which is now pointing downward, up and under the loop made by the left end. The tip of the right end should be pointing to the left.

Pull the right end through the loop in the back, making a bow. The right end will still be sticking down slightly.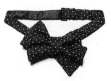

Pull lightly on both the left and right sides so they are parallel to the floor. Then pull again to adjust and tighten it.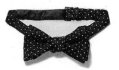

opposed to machine stitching (if it's tight and symmetrical, it's a machine).

"Buying a $50 tie, you also buy the exclusivity of design and the designer's name," Andersen concedes. With woven silk, the design is literally woven into the fabric, so the quality is better. Printed silk is more like painting on the fabric, so it may not hold as well. "If you buy a $10 silk tie, it may not be silk," warns Andersen. As with other clothes, Andersen says, Italian-made silk ties are among the best.

Walking through the tie section of any major men's store can overwhelm the senses. Just remember that there are basically just three things that set ties apart. They are:

1. Patterns. For years there were only stripes, solids, foulard (evenly spaced patterns covering the tie), club (small symbols repeated across a solid color), dotted, and paisley. Now the sky's the limit on patterns. The rule seems to be if it fits within the boundaries of the tie, it's fair game. "Pick patterns that match your personality," suggests Karpinski.

2. Knots. Know the three main knots and you'll be ready for anything. The Windsor is the largest; it's perfect for wide-spread collars. It needs a long tie. If your tie usually hangs too low, try this one. The half-Windsor fits regular-spread collars and should be used to add bulk to the look of lighter-weight silk ties. The four-in-hand looks good on tall men or men with round faces and works best with heavyweight fabrics. Use it with small-spread and tab collars.

3. Fabrics. Silk is the fabric of choice. Go high-end print or low-end woven and you won't go wrong. Silk ties hold colors better, tie better, and have a richer look and feel. Polyester "takes its raps aesthetically," says Andersen, "but there are no raps as far as wearability or performance go." Of the natural fabrics, cotton used to be considered a summer fabric, but now it's more associated with casual wear and is worn year-round. Wool, on the other hand, still tends to be seasonal, worn in fall and winter.

Here are a handful of other things to help you tie one on like a pro.

Make ends meet. There's nothing worse than a tie that doesn't reach down to a man's belt. "A short tie makes a man look like a rube who has just fallen off a turnip truck," Karpinski says. The ideal is for the narrow end and the wide to meet right at the buckle. But never let the narrow end be longer than the wide end.

Match width with width. Don't lose sleep worrying whether thin is in or wide is with it, suggests Andersen. The standard width of 3¾ inches is always in style, says menswear designer Alan Flusser. If there's any rule of thumb to follow, it's this: Wear wider ties with wider jacket lapels and thin ties with thin lapels to coordinate your look.

Buy quality ties. One way to tell if it's a quality tie is by flipping it over. In a good tie, the lining extends to the edge of the tie, says Andersen. Also look for hand stitching. Spread the wide end and if you see string hanging down, that's a sign that the tie was hand-sewn, which assures higher quality.

A good tie will last a very long time. If you think that the style has passed, don't throw it away. "Everything comes back again," Flusser says.

Let a pro clean it. If you keep confusing your tie for a bib, don't necessarily take matters into your own hands. If you spill water on your tie, first try a drop of water on the spot and then rub the fabric together over it, suggests Andersen. If it's a stain, anything beyond water—soap, for example—will do more harm than good. Spot remover will remove the color as well as the stain, causing permanent damage. "The best solution for almost all tie stains is to take it to the dry cleaner," Andersen advises.

Spike tie pins. As the casual look has become more the rule than the exception, tie pins have fallen out of favor, Karpinski says. Also, once you use a pin, you've put a hole in the tie. That forces you to wear the pin every time you wear that tie. Tie bars also are a thing of the past. If you feel you need to keep a tie in place, Karpinski suggests a tie chain, preferably of gold, which loops around the tie.

Sweaters

Pull the Wool over Your Eyes

It is, of course, a misnomer. The term *sweater* comes from the heavy blanket thrown over sweating thoroughbreds. On a man, the object of a sweater is not to make you sweat. It is, on the one hand, a functional accessory to keep you warmer and, on the other, a fashion accessory that can spiff up almost anything you wear, from jeans to a classic gray flannel suit. Sweaters not only serve multiple utilitarian purposes but also fulfill a variety of emotional needs. "They're the menswear equivalent of comfort food," says Peter Walsh of *DNR (Daily News Record)* and a self-professed sweater maven. "They're like familiar old friends. Even if it has holes in it, we'll keep an old sweater because we associate it with a time in our life and certain memories."

If Perry Como and Mr. Rogers are your role models, it's time to change the channel—and your sweater.

"Sweaters are a lot more versatile than people use them for," Walsh says. "A sweater can make an old suit look new. It can make a jacket and pair of slacks look like a completely different outfit. It can make you look very sophisticated—or very casual."

But because of their price tag—ranging from about $35 to $160 and up—sweaters "are not an impulse buy," notes Walsh.

Whether at the high end or low, there are some things that you can look for when you pick up a sweater that can immediately tell you if you're getting your money's worth. Before taking a sweater to the checkout line, check out these details.

Go from baaaa to worsted. One hundred percent worsted wool is best, says Patricia Auerbach, vice-president of sales for Tricots St. Raphael in New York City. This combing process gets rid of the little fibers, leaving the strongest and best part of the wool. The best wool comes from the moreno sheep of Uruguay, she adds.

Start with the finish. Look for a piece of fabric at the neck opening called the neck trim. There are two ways that it can be attached: looped with the same yarn that the sweater is made from or sewn by machine (also called merrowing). Looping is better. If it's machine-attached, it will come apart in laundering, Auerbach says.

Arm yourself. Turn the sweater inside out and look at the seam along the arm hole. Try to put your finger through where the arm attaches to the body. If it's loose, the sweater is poor-quality. It should be thick and closed, probably "fully fashioned," meaning that it has been knit from the bottom up, not cut from pieces.

Look for elasticity. A good sweater will have a thin band of elastic at the cuff of the sleeves and at the bottom of the sweater. Otherwise your cuffs will eventually be falling into your soup and your sweater will be down near your knees.

Pop a pill. Hold up the sweater and look at it at eye level. Does the surface have little balls? That's called pilling. If it looks that way before washing, it will look worse after, says Lenor Romano, director of design and merchandising for Pine State Knitwear in New York City, which dyes yarn and makes sweaters under a variety of their own and private labels.

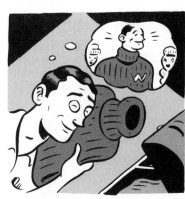

Go for blends, naturally. Synthetics added to natural fabrics ensure a longer life and better wear, Romano says. "Don't be afraid of acrylic and polyester," she says. "Five percent acrylic or Lycra gives cotton memory—something that plant life doesn't have."

The Classics

The Crew Neck ▶

This is your classic round-necked, stitched collar, which makes up about 90 percent of the sweaters sold. "This conservative but versatile look mixes and matches with impunity," says image consultant Ken Karpinski. It's a good outdoor-activities sweater because of the high closing of the collar. It goes well with a knit, button-down, or almost any other type of collar. In colder weather, wear it with a turtleneck shirt. It goes with dressy flannel or formal gabardine wool trousers, with a tweed, corduroy, or blazer jacket—anything with texture. What not to wear it with: pinstripe or chalk-stripe suits.

As for that question that we know haunts you every time you wear a crew neck sweater with a shirt, the answer is that the collar goes inside not outside the neck, says Lenor Romano of Pine State Knitwear, which dyes yarn and makes sweaters under a variety of its own and private labels.

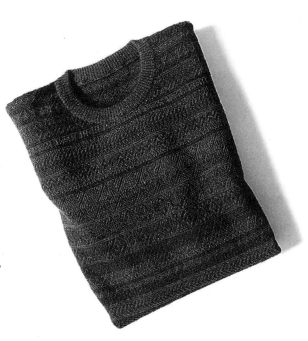

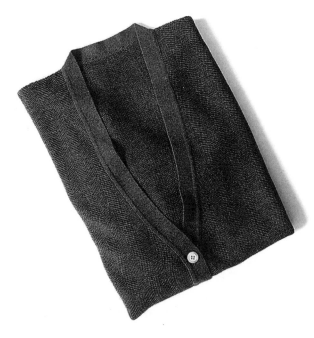

◀ The Cardigan

Named for the Earl of Cardigan, whose lesser accomplishment was leading the Charge of the Light Brigade, the classic version of this button-down has cable stitching (so named because it looks like a wound cable) and leather buttons and looks best when you're holding a pipe (you don't even have to smoke it for the effect). With or without sleeves, it can substitute for a sport jacket. In fact, many men, Karpinski among them, have kept a cardigan at work to change into during the day. "You'll still look dignified, but without the cumbersomeness of a sport jacket," he notes. Another plus: You don't muss your hair when you put it on. Want to know why you never button the bottom button? Some English monarch forgot to fasten it once, and his legions thought that he was making a fashion statement. To this day, mindlessly we follow suit.

The Turtleneck ▶

This is a fashionable look for the man who can pull it off. "It's more attractive on someone who has a neck than someone who doesn't," says Karpinski. (Football players, take note.) The traditional turtleneck has 4½ to 5 inches of material from the seam of the neck. Folded over, it comes to 2½ inches. For cold weather, this is the way to go. If you can afford the best wool, go for moreno. Other wools cause too much itching for sensitive necks. Or go with a non-itch cotton turtleneck. It is generally a great outdoor cold-weather sweater or for under sport jackets and even suits. A variation is the mock turtleneck, a shorter version for those of us who don't like all that weight around our necks. The mock, in fine wool or knit silk, is dressy enough to match with a high-priced suit.

◀ The V-Neck

Like the crew, this sweater is conservative and flexible. It is equally appropriate on Casual Friday or with a shirt and tie under a sport jacket or suit, especially in the sleeveless style. But, says Karpinski, this sweater looks better in more ranges of fabrics and patterns than the crew neck—from argyle and plaid to cashmere, wool, and wool blends. Avoid wearing a turtleneck shirt with a V-neck sweater, he adds. Because of the opening at the neck, this is not necessarily a utility sweater for deep winter but is ideal for early fall or spring.

Never wear a V-neck without a shirt "unless you have the pecs and lats to back it up," says Peter Walsh of *DNR (Daily News Record)* and a self-professed sweater maven.

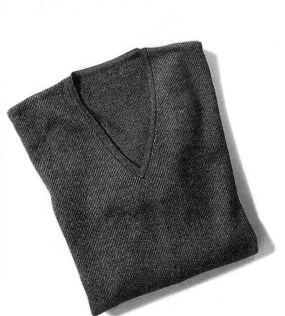

The Three-Buttoned Polo Neck ▶

Okay, so we snuck in something a bit more modern than classic. But, predicts Walsh, this look will become "a new classic before too long." The three-button polo has a regular shirt collar and buttons down to mid-chest. This works very well with a layered look—over a shirt, a turtleneck, or T-shirt.

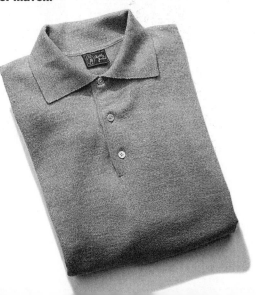

Outdoor Clothing

Coats for All Seasons

In theory, outerwear is meant to keep you dry and warm. But in real life, it serves another purpose: to project an image. Are you Humphrey Bogart (trench), Marlon Brando (leather), or Gordon Gekko (long, wool overcoat)? Or are you, in the words of Yvon Chouinard, founder of Patagonia, the outdoor clothing and equipment manufacturer, a "fun hog"—a guy who intends to be outside no matter what the weather (and wears rugged, multi-zippered, high-tech outerwear to tell the world as much)?

The truth is that a man of style should be equipped to be any and all of these. Plan on having at least three overcoats in the closet: one wool overcoat, a raincoat with a zip-out lining, and a warmer-weather jacket, maybe made of sheepskin or leather, says Michael Skidmore, vice-president of couture clothing and sportswear for Barney's New York in New York City.

Like much else in men's clothing, there is not a whole lot of diversity in choice when it comes to coat styles. But that doesn't mean your wool overcoat will be appropriate for a lifetime. "While there are many classic coat styles, each has gone through many changes in the past few years," Skidmore says. "Coats are shorter, slimmer, and have less cumbersome silhouettes than they used to."

What You Need

A coat serves a third function beyond warmth and image: clothing protection. And if you move in and out of buildings all day, you want one piece

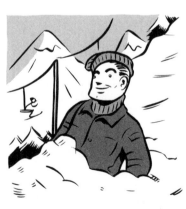

that you can take off and put back on easily but that is still heavy enough to protect you from rain, snow, and wind. Here's what to look for in the three main types of coats.

The Trench Coat

The classic trench coat, designed by Thomas Burberry, is more synonymous with Bogey than the World War I soldiers it was designed to dress. With epaulets (shoulder flaps), buckle cuffs, and a regulation-tan color, the trench is still a must-have for many men.

"A trench coat protects an investment, namely, an expensive suit," advises Ron Simcich, area manager of Troutman's Emporium in Tacoma, Washington. So if you go shopping for one but forget to bring a sport jacket, be sure to borrow one. The trench coat should fit comfortably over the jacket and cover most of your pants.

What else? The sleeves should be long enough to hide your jacket and shirt, and should have cuffs with buckles that tighten to keep out wind and rain. A collar that can turn up will protect your neck, while a yoke on the back allows water to slide off the coat so that it doesn't get soaked. Likewise, the pockets should have covers to prevent water from dripping inside. ("But no coat can replace an umbrella," Simcich says.)

To take a trench coat into the cold winter months, buy one with a removable lining. "And while there is usually a belt around the waist, never buckle it," Simcich says. "Instead, tie it casually around your waist, being careful to keep it loose enough to not wrinkle your clothes."

Although trench coats protect you from rain, they still have to be protected from water. Be sure to have them dry-cleaned. "Detergent can break down the chemicals that make the coat water-repellent," explains Simcich. "Dry cleaning will also keep the lines of the coat neat."

The Overcoat

Usually made of wool, the overcoat has little ornamentation other than buttons and a suit-style collar, and drapes down to below the knee. "Anyone who wears a jacket and tie to work is a good candidate for a traditional overcoat," says image consultant Ken Karpinski. A more luxurious—and considerably more expensive—option is a coat made from cashmere, a wool that comes from the cashmere goat, originally from Kashmir, India, says Karpinski. Overcoats tend to come in traditional colors: navy, gray, camel, black, or tweed. As for styles, they vary in subtle ways (see "Topcoats" on page 108).

Finally, you can consider a wrap coat, which has a wide, sash belt but no buttons, lending it a comfortable and opulent look, no matter what the fabric. "Big coats are less in style these days," Skidmore says. "You don't want to look as if you're wearing a bathrobe."

It is urban chic to wear a wool overcoat with casual clothes, such as jeans and a T-shirt, and if you can pull off the look, fine. But keep your best overcoat for your most formal occasions, Skidmore advises.

The Leather Jacket

A leather jacket makes a bold, maverick statement. But let's remember that although Brando wore a motorcycle jacket in *The Wild One*, he also wore jeans with cuffs—wide cuffs—in the movie. So you only want to take this imitation thing so far.

Now, black or brown? "Black dresses up clothes, even if it's a motorcycle jacket," Simcich says. "Brown is a more casual look." An even

Accessories Make the Man

Overcoats don't vary much. But the accessories can vary widely. Here are some guidelines for choosing gloves and scarves.

- **Gloves. Leather is your best bet, says Ron Simcich of Troutman's Emporium. "And if it's going to be really cold, make sure that the gloves have a lining to keep you warm because leather doesn't help on that front." As for color, simply match your coat. "Although if you're wearing a blue coat, your gloves should be cordovan, which is a burgundy leather," he says.**

- **Scarves. While you can't catch a cold from having a cold neck, it's not exactly comfortable either, so throw some warm cloth around your throat. "A scarf should be long enough to wrap around your neck twice without coming undone," Simcich says. "You can also tuck it into your collar."**

You have lots of options with scarves. A solid-colored coat looks great with a patterned scarf. Paisley, checks, and other patterns add excitement to dark blue or black. If you're wearing a coat that has a print such as herringbone, try a scarf that picks up one of the colors in the pattern. For a bolder look, wear a solid-colored scarf in a contrasting color, such as red.

better suggestion might be to hold up both coats against your skin and try to determine, or have someone in the store determine, which color is more flattering. "It's mostly just a matter of taste," Simcich says. "Although sometimes brown looks like you're not trying so hard to look cool."

As for rain and snow, it's a myth that they will hurt your jacket. "We get lots of rain here in Washington, and I wear my leather jacket all the time," says Simcich. "I waterproof it twice a year to keep it in good shape because it is an expensive investment."

While it's fine to wear a leather jacket, it is not okay to wear a leather coat. They are rarely in good taste, Simcich and Karpinski agree.

The Great Outdoors

"We build gear for a specific use," says Steve Rogerson, spokesman for Patagonia, an outdoor clothing and equipment manufacturer. "And although climbers, mountaineers, skiers, and surfers have different needs, in the end they all want to stay, for the most part, dry and warm.

"The first thing to do is ask yourself if the storm is going to be raging inside or outside," advises Rogerson. In other words, are you trying to protect yourself from elements of cold and wet, or are you going to be sweating so much during your sport that underneath your clothes you're going to create a raging furnace of perspiration?

"Synthetics have changed the way that we can enjoy outdoor activities," says Rogerson, who grew up sailing. "Being on the water used to mean being wet and cold, but not any more." Today, we can stay out longer

Topcoats

The Balmacaan

Single-breasted, with wide sleeves that extend to the neckline (called raglan)

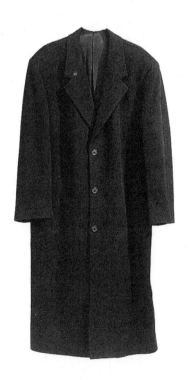

The Chesterfield

A more formal coat of dark gray and usually double-breasted with a velvet collar

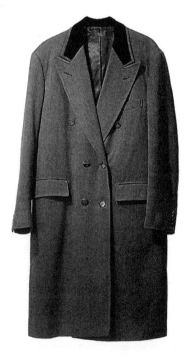

and be more comfortable.

No matter what your outdoor activity, think layers. "Start with a synthetic layer, such as Capilene, one that will wick away the perspiration," Rogerson says. "Whatever you do, stay away from cotton." Cotton gets wet and cold from your sweat, and that moisture will stay trapped next to your skin.

Your next layer should provide some insulation, spreading out your body heat and helping to dry the wet layer underneath it. A good suggestion is pile or fleece, which is lighter than wool. You also can go with down,

although it must be covered by a waterproof shell and can sometimes be "puffy," which cuts down on your ability to move freely.

Down-stuffed jackets have an aesthetic problem as well. "Anything with down is going to really bulk you up, which isn't attractive," remarks Simcich. "So stay away from that old ski jacket."

Finally, advises Rogerson, go for protection from the elements, specifically wind and water. "Ideally," he says, "your outer shell should have some sort of ventilation, continuing to help your skin breathe."

The Trench Coat

Raincoat that is traditionally tan and boasts its military past with epaulets, neck closures, and buckle cuffs

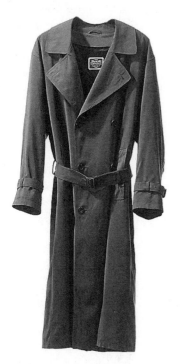

Classic Single-Breasted

Works on any body type; the long vertical line has a slight slimming effect

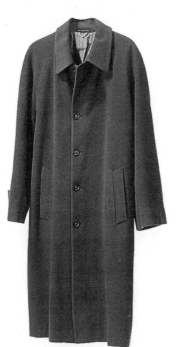

Classic Double-Breasted

A more formal look, especially in darker colors, such as navy and black

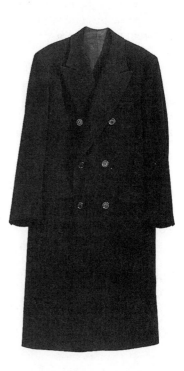

Underwear

Style That Doesn't Show

Somehow, it's hard to imagine that this was what the Founding Fathers had in mind when they cooked up that Freedom of the Press idea. There was President Bill Clinton, on MTV, being asked whether he wore boxers or briefs. And the funniest thing about it was that nobody was surprised when he confessed to being a briefs guy. Heck, few would have been surprised if he had unzipped on the spot to show off a snazzy pair of leopard-print Jockeys. But behind all the silliness lies an interesting question: What *can* you tell about a man from his choice in underwear?

Everything, says Ross E. Goldstein, Ph.D., a psychologist and president of Generation Insights, a consulting company in San Francisco. "When it comes to style, underwear may very well be the real window to the soul," Dr. Goldstein says. "They're one of the last bastions of self-expression. A person with real style leaves no stone unturned. There are always opportunities to express yourself, even in the most seemingly mundane ways."

And let's face it: Clothing doesn't get much more mundane than underwear.

"Boxers historically were what your father wore. I think briefs are more popular with Baby Boomer men because they have become another way for them to hold on to their youthfulness. Whereas wearing boxers, with younger men, like the Generation X and younger, has become a fashion statement unto itself."

Boxers or Briefs?

Of course, most men aren't worried about making a

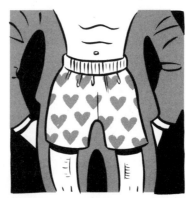

fashion statement with their underwear. Indeed, one Fruit of the Loom survey showed that just 26 percent of men prefer colored or patterned underwear. As far as most men are concerned, undershorts—and T-shirts, for that matter—serve two vital purposes: They keep you warm, and they keep you dry. That's why most underwear is made of cotton. As the world's most widely used fiber, cotton provides good ventilation. Plus, it absorbs moisture and is soft and easy to care for. Some upscale underwear features mercerized cotton, which has been stretched and immersed in harsh chemicals to make it softer. When cotton is blended with other fabrics for underwear, it's often a minority blend of synthetic polyester or stretchy Lycra.

Boxers earn 25 percent of the dollars that men spend on underwear, and sales have been growing in double digits for the past few years. But unlike the boxers that you probably remember your old man wearing, these come in all sorts of colors and patterns, from military white to sultry silk. "With the influx of younger consumers, especially in the boxer market, we're seeing underwear that's different from what your grandfather wore," says Jeanie Wilson of Sara Lee Knit Products in Winston-Salem, North Carolina, director of marketing for Hanes underwear. "Today it's a fashion statement, an expression of style. It's like buying a tie."

Moreover, boxers look good on anybody. "Boxers as a style are flattering to almost any shape or size," says image consultant Ken Karpinski. They're also popular as loungewear, outerwear, and as shorts for women.

All that said, most men are still wearing briefs. They're comfortable and they're preferred by men who—how shall we say?—aren't at ease with the feeling of genitalia freedom that boxers afford. Once again, there are scores of styles, colors, and patterns to choose from these days.

"The basic military-issue

underwear or the run-of-the-mill briefs that you grew up with are very, very unappealing given what's out there today," says Sam Baker, president, chief executive officer, and chief designer at Male Power LTD, an exotic underwear manufacturer in Bay Shore, New York.

If you can't decide between boxers or briefs, there's a hybrid called boxer-briefs. They're shorter, tighter-fitting boxers that combine the best of both worlds.

Under Wraps

Here's how to look stylish from the inside out.

Be fit to a T. T-shirts are necessities in the business world, so don't even think of leaving for work without one. Undershirts absorb moisture, a plus when you're giving a presentation and don't want your audience to see proof of how nervous you are. They also protect your outer shirts from sweat stains. If you are wearing a shirt made of sheer fabric, wear a classic T-shirt, not a sleeveless undershirt.

Never show the world what style T-shirt you're wearing, unless you're doing an underwear commercial. If you're wearing a pullover golf shirt, stick with V-neck style Ts. Otherwise, standard crew necks (round collars) are good for all occasions. Single-pocket colored Ts—black, maroon, tan—are also good for a stylish layered look with chinos, or by themselves with khakis or new blue jeans for very casual affairs.

Slide on the silks. Silk boxers are the tuxedos of undergarments. An investment of $15 to $40 gets you luxurious underwear with the look and feel of elegance. Plus they're enormously comfortable.

Go long, John. Thermal underwear, or long johns, trap heat and keep you toasty when the rest of the world is an ice cube. Long johns

---

Underwear, Outerwear

In what could be one of the most brilliant marketing schemes in underwear history, designers have widened their waistbands, printed their names in supersize letters, and featured ads with models proudly showing their Skivvies. The result? A new fashion trend. Even in Japan, where so-called Ko-Gals (teenage girls) are shocking their elders by baring their briefs and boxers.

"That look is important to young people, and they're advertising for the designer at the same time," says Jeanie Wilson of Sara Lee Knit Products. "Underwear once was something that you didn't talk about, but it's almost a part of your outerwear collection today."

Which leads us to ask: Why?

So we asked a psychologist.

"When people are younger, they're more influenced by external sources. They try on different selves, different identities, often with dramatic shifts," says Dr. Ross E. Goldstein of Generation Insights. "Some experimentation is normal, whether it's with the hair or underwear."

So for the most part, if your kid's wearing his BVDs in plain sight, it's probably nothing to worry about. If your boss is, well, that's another story.

---

also wick moisture away from your body. In addition to white, two-piece lumberjack sets, there are high-performance suits that run up to $60.

Try nifty novelties. Animal prints. Floral prints. Glow-in-the-dark prints. Thongs. They're out there. But are they for you?

"If you're confident and sure of your identity, you can wear anything," Baker says. "My friends say that their wives would never let them wear erotic underwear, but it's after they get divorced that they come to me. They find that erotic underwear makes them feel sexier. It says something about their personality."

Jewelry

All That Glitters Is Not Sold

Men have been buying jewelry forever. The difference now is that increasing numbers are buying it for themselves—not their wives and girlfriends. But it's not like your average corporate executive is going to show up for the next board meeting flashing ostentatious baubles on his fingers like Ringo Starr, or layers of gold chains around his neck like Mr. T. (We pity the fool who would do that. His future would be about as bright as, well, Mr. T's.) No, men are going for a far more subtle approach.

"We found that it isn't the jewelry itself that men object to but the styles that they've been offered over the years," says Andrea Menezes, marketing director for H. Stern Jewelers in New York City. Men tend to prefer textured and matte metals (as opposed to shiny). And this isn't like the Olympics: They're going for the silver as well as the gold. "Men like and look best in pieces that are bold-looking but also plain," Menezes says.

In general, men should stick to strong and unornamented metals, although gems and stones are an option, provided that they're discreet and not very shiny, she says.

Rings and Things

If you're thinking about investing in precious metals, here are some things to keep in mind.

Pay the price. "Jewelry is an investment," Menezes says. "However, it's more about building an image than about putting money in the bank." Good jewelry, she adds, should come with a guarantee

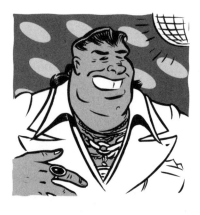

regarding the quality of the metal as well as the class of any stones. And the jeweler should explain how often he will need to clean the piece and check its settings. Once a year is usually enough.

Choose your own. You're happily married, but your wedding band just seems to rub you the wrong way. Allergic to marriage? No, it's more likely that you let her pick out the rings. Don't make the same mistake twice. "Men won't wear anything that isn't comfortable," says Menezes, "and the only way to tell if a piece is comfortable is to try it on before purchasing it."

Design your own. Don't assume that what sits in the jeweler's case is all that he has to offer. The jewelry shown is just a general idea of the possibilities. "You may like the look of one ring but find that another one fits more comfortably," Menezes says. "Tell the jeweler that, because very often they can mix and match styles. So try on pieces that you don't like, just to see if they have elements that you find comfortable."

Start small. If you're going to buy a piece of jewelry for yourself, Menezes advises starting with a ring. "It's the most discreet piece and very acceptable in society because of wedding bands, class rings, and the like," she says.

Rings, however, are the most difficult pieces to fit. Menezes says that you want to be sure that you can close your hand easily, so look for rings with a shank (the part of the ring that sits between your fingers) that isn't too high or wide. Also, many rings come with a "comfort fit," which means the inside of the band is curved to give your finger some breathing space.

Brace yourself. Do you like your ring and want to get something to keep it company? "A second-choice purchase might be a bracelet," says Menezes. "Anything after that requires a lot of self-assurance." One guideline: Don't mix metals. If your ring is silver, find a complementary silver necklace or bracelet.

If you are going to wear a bracelet or necklace, consider something thin and perhaps even personal, such as a small religious medal that will probably hang well below your shirt collar.

You know what look you're *not* going for (see Mr. T, above). "To wear jewelry well," explains Menezes, "remember that it is not an outfit accessory. It's a statement about who you are. You don't want to become a walking window for jewelry. Instead, you want the jewelry to reflect your own taste and sense of style."

Keep Watch

Odds are that even the most conservative guy already is wearing one article of jewelry. You notice, across the polished oak desk of the boardroom, that the president of the company wears a watch that seems to be made from the thinnest sliver of gold you've ever seen. Or you observe that your diving instructor wears a watch that doesn't just tell time but measures depth and speed as well. Watch, and you'll learn a lot about most men.

"The kind of watch you wear determines what kind of guy you are," says Susie Watson, advertising and public relations director for Timex in Middlebury, Connecticut. "President Bill Clinton wore our Ironman watch to his first Inaugural Ball, which was an incredible statement of casualness. It now hangs in the Smithsonian next to Abraham Lincoln's gold pocket watch."

Picking out a watch involves asking yourself just a few easy questions.

"Despite all the options out there, your first concern is price. What can you afford?" Watson says.

An expensive watch, Watson says, usually reflects the materials used to make it. "If you're spending thousands of dollars for a watch, it's probably made of precious metals, such as gold, silver, or platinum. It's the ingredients that have the value, not its timekeeping abilities," she says.

In fact, Watson says, mid-priced and low-end watches often keep better time than expensive watches. "You have to wind a Rolex and other watches of that class," Watson says. "But other watches are made with quartz, and from the point of view of accuracy, one quartz watch is usually as good as the next." The battery in a quartz watch should last from three to five years, she says.

Meanwhile, mid-priced watches, such as Tag Heuer, and low-cost watches, such as Timex, have fewer distinguishing qualities. "Watches that cost $500 to $600 are usually made of the same things as those under $100," Watson says. "When you're choosing between those, you're choosing between brand name and style."

So, now it's time to pick out your watch. "What do you need?" asks Watson. "What do you want? An alarm? A stopwatch? Do you want an analog or digital face? In other words, don't buy what you don't need." (And, by the way, in the world of watches, stopwatches are now known as chronographs.)

Even low-end watches can be of varying quality. "Check out the leather," advises Watson. "Is the stitching strong? Is the finish consistent?"

For many men, a watch is the only defining piece of jewelry they own, so design is the number one thing they look for. "Your watch should work with your clothes," Watson says. "A black strap, which is dressy and these days kind of outdated, doesn't fit a plaid shirt or casual clothes." Brown leather straps and sport watches are the biggest percentage of the market.

That doesn't mean that you should pack away your great-grandfather's timepiece. As with any jewelry, a truly fine watch is a work of art. So wear a pocket watch at appropriate times (with a vest that has a pocket for one), or keep it in the pocket of your jeans, without the chain attached. A gift from your family is perhaps the most stylish watch of all.

Shoes

Stepping Out in Style

There's a lot of pressure on your feet. And it's not from being stuck under that big bag of bulk you call your body.

"Shoes can often be the most obvious sign of a man's sense of style and social position," says menswear designer Alan Flusser.

It's one thing to hear that from a man, but when a woman talks, men sit up and listen: "No doubt about it, shoes give women a quick insight into a man's personality, his self-esteem, his sexiness," confides image consultant Carolyn Gustafson.

Surprisingly, it's not the style or price tag of his footwear that reveals the soul of a man. Often it's how well he maintains them. Eighty-eight percent of the respondents to a survey said that they form positive impressions of people based on well-maintained shoes. "If the shoes are polished, if the heels aren't run down, if the laces are not frayed, and if the soles don't have holes—this all tells me that a man knows how to take care of himself, that he's responsible and probably dependable," says Gustafson.

Adds Debbi Karpowicz, Boston-based author of *I Love Men in Tasseled Loafers*, "A man who cares for and protects his footwear will do the same for you."

So since the people we care most about care most about how well we care for our shoes, let's fill that order first before we try on a couple of styles.

The Well-Maintained Shoe

For the man who protects his wallet as carefully as he protects his stylish reputation,

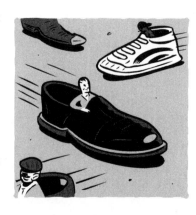

keeping your shoes in good shape is a wise investment, says Gail Sundling, president of the Delmar Bootery in Albany and Delmar, New York, and a member of the board of directors of Shoe SMARTS (that's Shine, Maintain, and Repair Those Shoes), a Baltimore-based organization representing shoe repair professionals. "The upkeep of your shoes is a fraction of the cost of buying a new pair," she says. Here are a couple of things that she suggests to make your shoes last longer.

Heels, boy. That's a recommendation, not a command. A new pair of heels can uplift the look of a downtrodden pair of shoes. The average wear time is about six months, depending on use and the material, before they start looking funky. A combination of rubber and leather will give you both durability and a good look. Rubber heels are a third of the cost and more durable, though they look like . . . rubber. A pair of heels costs $9 to $16. If you want to add a couple of months to the life of your heel, spend $1 to $2 on heel savers, those crescent-shaped pieces that attach to the back of heels.

Soothe your soles. There are as many grades of leather soles as there are grades of meat in a market. Grade 1 is filet mignon. Grade 5 is ground chuck. The good ones will last up to two years. A pair of Grade 1 soles plus heels together (that's called full soles) will set you back from $38 to $45. For Grade 5 full soles, subtract about $8. For an additional $14 to $17 you can get a protective sole, a long thin rubber-made piece that doesn't affect the flexibility of the shoe but will extend the life of the sole about three times. Half-soles (minus the heels) cost $25 to $28.

Grow a shoe. Shoe trees can stretch the life of a shoe. "I don't care if you spend $40 or $400 on a pair of shoes," says Sundling. "The thing that will kill them is perspiration." At night the perspiration

Sock It to Me

Archaeologists have discovered knitted socks in Egyptian tombs dating back more than 2,000 years. More recently, socks very much resembling those from Egypt were discovered behind your washing machine, along with the rest of the stray singles that you've been missing.

If you're a typical guy, your interest in socks is limited to three things: how warm they keep you, how well they fit you, and whether they match your outfit. The typical guy buys about 11 pairs of socks a year, says Sid Smith, president of the National Association of Hosiery Manufacturers in Charlotte, North Carolina. Almost 60 percent of them are bought in a discount department store, and we pay an average of $1.45 per pair.

For warmth, stick with the natural fabrics of cotton and wool. They insulate better, absorb foot moisture better, and dry faster, says Smith. The synthetics will give you strength and flexibility but not much protection against the cold.

When it comes to matching your outfit, the first rule of thumb is never wear black socks with shorts. The second is that red socks don't work, says image consultant Ken Karpinski, not coincidentally the author of *Red Socks Don't Work*. The third, he notes, regardless of color or pattern, is that a gentleman should never reveal his hairy shins to the world. Short socks are right up there with short ties in Karpinski's list of male fashion sins. Other than that, he recommends mixing up your styles. Solids every day are boring. Venture out. Try such patterns as bird's-eye, nail's head, cable-stitch, herringbone, even argyle.

As for getting the right fit, Smith says that three variables—the kind of yarn, the kind of knitting machine, and the knit construction—can affect how well a pair hugs your footsies. Pay attention to the manufacturers' fitting suggestions. Meanwhile, the National Association of Hosiery Manufacturers suggests following these standard guidelines.

Shoe size	Sock size
4½–5½	9½
6–6½	10
7–8	10½
8½–9	11
9½–10	11½
10½–11	12
11½	12½
12–12½	13
13–14	14
14½–16	15
16½–18	Try a small duffel bag

evaporates and rots the shoe from the inside out. Cedar shoe trees will air out the shoe because the wood has open pores, letting the leather dry and breathe. They also help maintain the original shape of the shoe, avoiding that elf-like curling action at the toes. If you use them in your sneakers, Sundling adds, you could add up to two years to their life. You can buy a cedar tree from a shoe repair professional for $11 to $45.

Blow your shoe horn. Those little plastic or metal gadgets that accumulate in your sock drawer really do serve a purpose. They save the counter, the protective piece at the back that stabilizes the structure of the shoe. That, in turn, supports your ankles, your knees, and your hips and eventually helps keep your whole body erect. "When you step into the shoe without a horn, you crush the counter and the shoe becomes worthless," Sundling says.

Sport a shiner. Keeping them shined is the fundamental rule of well-kept shoes. Not only will they look better—Would you go to a formal affair with a dirty face?—but the polish protects them. Use a polish with a wax base. Sundling is partial to creams or paste, but not the liquid or spray-ons. You can guard leather suede or fabric shoes against the elements by using nonsilicone water and stain protector.

You're a Shoe-In

Now for the easy part: what kind of dress shoes to wear. It's easy because "the choices in footwear are very basic," says Michael J. Kormos, president of Footwear Market Insights, a Nashville-based company that analyzes footwear trends. "There are maybe a dozen

If the Shoe Doesn't Fit . . .

Put your foot down when the footwear doesn't fit right, says William Van Pelt, D.P.M., a past president of the American Academy of Podiatric Sports Medicine. "Men constantly buy the wrong shoes for the wrong reasons. And it's contributing to a lot of foot problems out there, like calluses, corns, blisters, bunions, and heel spurs," he says. One way to make sure that you get a good fit is to know the shape of your foot, as opposed to your size. Feet come in three shapes, or lasts: straight, curved, and standard. Men with flat arches should wear shoes with straight lasts. High arches need curved lasts. And normal arches feel best in standard lasts.

Here's a quick way to figure out your last. Sitting down, place your bare right foot on a piece of paper on the floor and trace its outline. A straight line from toe to heel is a flat arch. An extremely curved line is a high arch. A standard arch is somewhere in between the two. To figure out if a shoe has the kind of last you need, turn it over and examine the sole for the curve that most looks like your foot's.

To get the best fit, your shoe should be three-quarters of an inch longer than your foot while standing, says Robert Schwartz, president of Eneslow, a specialty shoe fitting company in New York City; a certified pedorthist (a person who fits shoes and related devices to help ease foot discomfort or disorders); and past president of the Pedorthic Footwear Association. That way, there's room for your foot to spread as the day wears on. Also, the more support a shoe offers, the better for your feet. So

variations on three styles that have been around for many years: the wing tip, the cap-toe, and the loafer."

look for shoes with more structure and body, with arch supports under the balls of your feet "so that you feel like there's some substance under foot," he adds.

Heed these other tips to keep your toes in tip-top shape.

Size up your feet regularly. Feet grow, too. A man's feet grow longer and wider as he ages, Dr. Van Pelt explains. That's why it's a good idea to have your feet measured every time you buy a new pair. You should stand when your feet are measured because they lengthen and widen under the weight of your body.

Trust your feet. If you try on a pair of shoes in your size and they feel uncomfortable, don't buy them just because you think they should fit. "A good shoe must feel comfortable immediately upon putting it on," says John Stollenwerk, president and owner of Allen-Edmonds Shoe Corporation in Port Washington, Wisconsin, one of the top high-end American shoe manufacturers. "Don't believe a salesman who says, 'This will stretch, or put pads here or there.' " Try another size. Or another style. Or another brand. Think of shoes like snowflakes. Because of the imperfections of manufacturing, no two are exactly alike. And don't think that enough wear will eventually *make* them fit. Shoes that are too small when you buy them will be too small in the next millennium.

Shop late. If somebody had been standing on you all day, you'd start to flatten and spread, too. Shop at the end of the day to make sure that the shoes will fit all day—and night.

at the thought of Imelda Marcos's shoe closet, most men on average own about eight pairs. We buy an average of three to four pairs a year, says Kormos. Every two years we may toss some out. "It's the characteristic of shoes that people don't throw them away," he says. "No ones knows why not." It could be the average price that we pay for a pair: $61.

Here are the main styles and what occasions they're most appropriate for.

• The oxford. This is your basic lace-up shoe, sporting three to six sets of eyelets. The plain-toe variety has no lines, no extra leather, no frills. The cap-toe has an extra layer of leather at the toe end of the shoe. Plain or with a perforated or medallion decoration, this shoe is the "dressiest business shoe you can wear," says image consultant G. Bruce Boyer.

• The wing tip. This is a fully brogued (meaning that there's added leather for protection) oxford. In black, it's for business attire, says Boyer; in brown, it can be worn with dressy sportswear. Because they are a little more ornate, they're usually considered less formal than plain-toe oxfords, adds Boyer. "But they still reflect a more traditional style."

• The slip-on. This would include the dressier plain slip-on, the tasseled variety, and the collegiate-looking penny loafer. The dressy sort, like expensive Gucci's, can be worn with business suits, or with dressy casual wear. The tasseled loafer is a "good all-around multipurpose shoe," says Boyer. It's appropriate for business, upscale casual, or very casual scenes. The brown penny loafer, sometimes called the weejun, should be worn only in casual situations—never with a business suit.

Even with those few varieties, it appears that most men still like to keep their choices simple. While some women might have drooled

• The monk strap. No, it's not an athletic supporter for priests. This slip-on shoe has a plain tip with a buckled strap that crosses the instep. It can be worn formally or with a business suit in black or dark brown, or with informal wear that's more dressy. Wearing it with casual attire "would be a mistake," adds Boyer.

In the past 20 years, another category has made great strides in popularity. Casual dress shoes now make up about 16 percent of the total number of men's shoes sold. Ergo, Rockport, New Balance, Reebok, and dozens of imitators all make them. The idea is simple: Use soles of the type found on most sneakers (one layer for traction, one for cushion, made from a blown, spongy, white rubber called ethylvinyl acetate), top them with leather or suede or anything but canvas, and you have a shoe that looks—and feels—good in the boardroom, at the barbecue party, or for the 20-block walk through Manhattan.

"Casual shoes are an outgrowth of the popularity of the running craze," says George Dietel, vice-president of men's shoes marketing at Rockport, the company based in Marlboro, Massachusetts,

Are You a Heel?

If you've ever wondered how and why gals fall for the guys they fall for, Debbi Karpowicz, author of *I Love Men in Tasseled Loafers*, advises: Look down, young man.

"There may be 50 ways to leave your lover but only one way to judge him," says Karpowicz. "I go right to his shoe rack. Any man can go out and buy a gray pinstripe suit and look the same as any other man. One of the few ways that a man can express his individuality is in his accessories. And—I'm not sure exactly why—but, to a woman, shoes say everything that she needs to know about a man's personality and his economic status."

We asked Karpowicz to share some of her footnotes on what men's shoes say about them. Here is her response (remember that this is just one woman's opinion).

- *Penny loafers:* "Simply marvelous. This bud's for me. Likes commitment, holding hands, and Harry Winston jewelry."
- *Tassel loafers:* "This man is the Rolls-Royce of relationships. Close encounters of the best kind."

that now is the number one casual shoe manufacturer. Running led to the walking-for-fitness boom, which led to design innovations in what

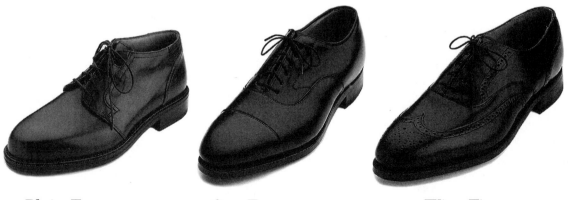

Plain-Toe   Cap-Toe   Wing Tip

- **Wing tips:** "The shoes have no appendage—need I say more? Still wears Old Spice and his high school ring."
- **Cowboy boots:** "Watch your step. Tacky and likely to wear a fake Rolex watch with an imitation gold-nugget wristband."
- **Mid-calf boots:** "Macho men who will step on you and forbid you to talk to other men—even priests."
- **Construction boots:** "Boot him. He probably reads Hustler."
- **Monk straps:** "Awful! Yech! Hand him his walking papers."
- **Earth shoes:** "He probably still wears Nehru jackets and leisure suits. Give him some granola and get rid of him."
- **Sandals:** "He's callous, usually has dirty clothes and hair, and wears a weird beard. The worst offenders wear Birkenstocks, especially with socks in public."
- **Topsider boat shoes:** "Leaves a yacht to be desired."
- **Virgin vinyl and/or white shoes:** "No comment."

the rest of the time. The industry responded.

"These shoes have revolutionized the shoe industry," says Bill Boettge, president of the National Shoe Retailers Association. "And they fit in perfectly with the whole casual swing of men's clothing."

Of course, there are other shoe types. The white buck. The deck shoe. The chukka or desert boot. The moccasin. The sandal in all its infinite variety. And the good old cowboy boot, which experiences waves of popularity, depending on the ups and downs of country music. And then there are the also-rans, or, in this case, the barely walkeds. That is, the fad shoes that drag their feet through the fashion world from time to time: the Earth shoes of the 1970s; the blue suede shoes of the 1950s made famous by Elvis Presley; the Hush Puppies, which we've heard are making a comeback; and the wooden clogs, which we borrowed from the Dutch and luckily returned to them shortly after we developed serious bunions. Men who wear these shoes are either bold enough to march to the beat of a different drummer or stupid enough to follow just about anybody in front of them. Which are

became known as performance or fitness shoes. Once men got used to how comfortable shoes could feel, they came to expect that feel

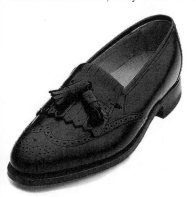 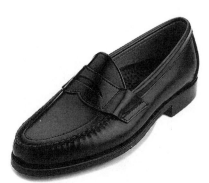 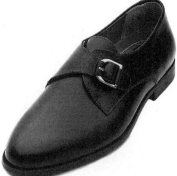

Tassel Loafer   Penny Loafer   Monk Strap

you? As they say, if the shoe fits . . .

If a man were to pick three pairs of the above styles that he'd get the most mileage out of, Dietel would recommend a pair of wing tips for dress, a pair of slip-on loafers in his favorite style, and a pair of comfortable casual walking shoes, the last two for either work or play.

One other style detail: color. In the old days—back before the 1970s—it was sort of like the old adage about Model T Fords: You had your choice of any color, as long as it was black. Now black is still the most popular—and versatile—color, especially in the dressy category, according to Dietel. But burgundy and brown have become players, too. In casual shoes, brown outsells black, while burgundy is number two and tan is number three.

"Burgundy makes a strong statement," adds Dietel. It goes with gray, navy, black, and tan. Tan also goes with any of the aforementioned, except black. If you want to push the envelope of your basic brown, try its modern variations: a color called espresso or another known as cognac British.

Boost Your Buying Power

If you know exactly what you're looking for, a discount shoe chain or department store is fine, suggests Boettge. "But at a specialty shoe store, you'll get a lot more information on what to wear with what and when."

If economics are your primary consideration, says Boettge, "dollar for dollar you can go to Payless and get good shoes for good value." However, if your feet are extremely wide or narrow and you have trouble finding a comfortable fit, or if you're on your feet all day—say, in retail or working construction—he recommends a specialty shoe store.

If you're one of the 4 to 7 percent of people who have serious feet problems, or if you think you might be, go to a certified

pedorthist, a specialist who fits shoes on such people.

Brand-name stores that carry only the shoes that they manufacture frequently offer just as good a deal as the department store down the street. "Prices are dictated by the competition," says Boettge. "Timberland or Florsheim don't want you to walk down to Macy's and find the same shoe for $10 less." And some brand-name stores also carry shoes that they don't make.

Another tip that Boettge offers for getting the biggest bang for your white bucks is to shop at factory outlets and deep-discount stores. "This is a good bet if you're not interested in the latest fashions but in quality and name brands," he says, though "finding irregular sizes there can be a challenge."

There are several ways to recognize a good shoe. John Stollenwerk of Allen-Edmonds Shoe Corporation shares some.

Look at the leather. Leather from a young calf is the best. It will last longer and resist cracking. Good natural calf's skin won't have scars or wrinkles or veins. It will be smooth and have a mirror finish. If it looks painted or varnished, it's a less-expensive leather.

Be a sole man. A good-quality sole is light tan. "Some manufacturers will paint the sole black to hide the blemishes," Stollenwerk says. The sole should be flexible. Bend it to find out.

Don't come unglued. Ask the salesman for shoes with soles that are hand-stitched to the upper, which Stollenwerk believes is better than cement-gluing. The stitching process is called Goodyear welting. "You can actually feel the stitching if you run your hand along the inside edge," he says. But to be sure, double-check with the salesman—and hope that he's trustworthy.

Study the stitch. Stitching should be neat, close to the edges of the shoe. The thread should be a white cotton.

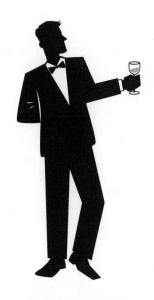

Part Four

Always in Style

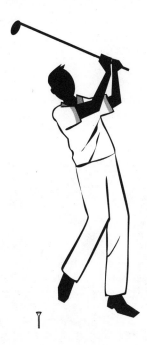

In the Bedroom

What to Wear with a Nightcap

At most places, the dress code is clear. At a restaurant? No shirt, no shoes, no service. At work? No tie, no jacket, no promotion.

Sartorial things in life are generally spelled out on a sign or in a book somewhere.

Except in the bedroom.

It may seem simple at first blush: Get naked. And get in bed. But like most things in life, it's more complicated than that. For example, what if you're spending the night in someone else's quarters for the first time? What if you're looking to jump-start your love life? What about loungewear? Cold nights and colder feet? And then there are all the tricky issues revolving around how to act and what to say. Being a stylish lover—now *there's* a goal worth pursuing.

Room for Style

Style in the bedroom is important. Not only are you sleeping there every night but also it's where your most intimate moments occur. Statistics show that one in three of us between the ages of 18 and 59 have sex twice a week or more. Another third "do the deed" at least a few times a month. One thing that you can bet on: What you wear and how you conduct yourself in the bedroom will have a direct impact on how often you have sex—and how much fun it is when you do.

"Men don't think about subtle sexy things, like what they wear to bed. We're conditioned to be fighters, not lovers," says Sam Baker, president, chief executive officer, and chief designer at Male Power LTD, an exotic underwear manufacturer in

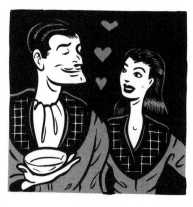

Bay Shore, New York.

That's sad, Baker adds, because "style matters so much in the bedroom. It's part of the mood. Underwear, lingerie, your bedroom eyes, everything you say or do in the bedroom perpetuates the feelings. It's your job to make the most of them, and clothing helps."

And we're not just talking sex. Your sleeping quarters also play host to a variety of activities: lounging, reading, deep discussion. When it comes to what you're wearing, the bedroom offers latitude to prove that your style sense doesn't end at the office.

"Men have always had it easier at this. We're beneficiaries of laxer dress standards and have more freedom," says Ross E. Goldstein, Ph.D., a psychologist and president of Generation Insights, a consulting company in San Francisco.

That's because there's a bit of a double standard between men and women when it comes to the dress code, including nighttime dress code. A man, for example, can wear boxers and a T-shirt to bed and be normal. A woman in boxers and a T-shirt, or in sweats and a sweatshirt, is frumpy.

Here's how to improve your image in the bedroom by wearing—and doing—the right stuff.

Be a man with a plan. What to wear in the bedroom depends largely on what you're planning to do. If you're spending the night at someone's house for the first time, or vice versa, you'll dress differently than if you're recovering from a back injury for two weeks. Think ahead and plan your nighttime wardrobe with as much forethought as your daytime outfit.

"Black socks and white baggy underpants aren't all that attractive at the end of a good date, but I suppose if you've gotten that far, you're home free," quips David Wolfe, creative director and chief trend forecaster at The Doneger

Group, a buying house and fashion forecasting firm in New York City. The question you might want to ponder is, Will there be a repeat performance?

Don't dis robes. Hugh Hefner you're not, and maybe you never want to be. But the old playboy is on to something when it comes to loungewear. Robes are comfortable. Any woman will tell you that the thin, cheap Kmart-type robe that you wore as a kid won't cut it. Nothing cuts it short of thick, luxurious, warm, and full-length. Good robes can cost $40 or more, but they'll last and are worth every penny. (And they'll look great on her, too.)

Climb in the ring. Forget those saggy, white briefs you've been wearing. "Aesthetics is very personal, of course, but a lot of women, especially younger women, think that boxers are sexy because they look good on different types of men," says Jeanie Wilson of Sara Lee Knit Products in Winston-Salem, North Carolina, director of marketing for Hanes underwear.

Bikini briefs are still worn by many men, and preference seems to be regional as well as personal. For example, Wilson says, Europeans tend to prefer bikini briefs and flashier colors in underwear. Our advice? Unless you have a body that can carry off Speedos on the beach, choose boxers. Preferably silk ones.

Get exotic—and erotic. Male Power LTD's line of exotic underwear, and others like it, are surefire style enhancers.

"A lot of this stuff is frowned upon by guys, but it works. Wearing exotic underwear makes you feel sexy," says Baker, whose product line includes underwear in animal prints, sheer material, fishnet, lace, thongs, G-strings, and novelties.

"Today, we're more open about these things. Exotic underwear is gift wrap for your lover. You're bringing her yourself in style," Baker says.

Smooth out the wrinkles. No matter what you're wearing, consider making it a cotton/polyester blend, suggests Wilson. Blends are popular choices for loungewear, underwear, and lingerie because they don't wrinkle easily,

guaranteeing a fresh-pressed look, even after your outfit's been under your suit all day.

Wear a sleek physique. Fitness and good health are always in fashion, and nothing looks better on a guy than well-toned muscles and low body fat. "Women talk about men's physical appearances these days—their bodies, shoulders, and butts," Wolfe says. "Women are looking at you more as a sex object and not as much for security, because they don't need that as much. And, hey, if you're in better shape, even cheaper clothes look good on you."

Shoot for silk and its ilk. Silk is "special-occasion" material in the bedroom. Silk boxers, silk pajamas, even silk sheets are famous for their luster and luxuriousness. If silk's too expensive, consider satin. Or "sand-washed" silk, which, after debuting in 1991, is nothing more than microdenier polyester treated with chemicals and roughed up by sand for a smooth, silky finish.

Decorate for love. Your bedroom's decor tells a woman a lot about you. Ditch those old, pilled sheets that you've been using for too long. Buy nice satin ones for the summer and warm, soft flannel ones for the winter. Invest in new pillows—easily camouflaged sex accessories—and stick a stool in a corner. It's a great shelf for books and papers and can come in handy for certain sex positions. Pay attention to music and lighting, too. A radio and/or CD or tape player should be the only electronic device on in your room if love is in the air. If you have a TV, make sure that it's off. The 11:00 o'clock news doesn't quite set the right mood. Lighting should come from candles, dimmer lights, even black lights near the headboard. (Black lights give you and your lover the appearance of a healthy tan, without the adverse side effects of tanning.)

Keep it clean. A clean, well-organized bedroom can make a big positive statement to that first-time visitor by showing that you respect yourself. It also is far better than the alternative. Do you want women to see clothes piled on the floor, closet doors open, shoes and magazines everywhere, an unmade bed?

At the Beach

Get in the Swim of Things

As Deputy Beach Chief of Volusia County Beaches for the Daytona Beach area in Florida, Joe Wooden has spent a quarter-century watching wave after wave of swimwear styles change like the tide.

"Culture goes through cycles, and what's hot on the beach is no exception," Wooden says. "When you're on the beach for so many years, you become acclimated to what you see. Nothing sticks out to me the way that it used to."

Wooden has seen swimsuit styles sink and swim. He's watched baggy trunks change to sheer microbriefs and then back to baggy trunks. He's watched suit bottoms widen and narrow, and seen throngs in thongs. He even remembers what sounds like beach blasphemy today: tanning contests.

"Remember those? In the 1970s, we'd have contests right here on the beach to see who could get the darkest," Wooden says. "No one thought about cancer. Your only protection was a little zinc oxide on your lips or nose, but only because you didn't want pain. Cancer had nothing to do with it."

Oh, how times have changed.

Looking Good While Wet

While some people still insist on sporting a native tan, most concede that being covered in cancerous melanomas is far from fashionable.

"The group still at the greatest risk is teenagers, especially females. Looks are so im-

portant to them," Wooden says. Grown men like yourself, however, are wiser, because "with age comes responsibility, and that includes your skin."

Suits have evolved, too. Just a century ago, you'd have seen beachgoing men in what looked like long johns. (Women had it worse; their outfits included full-length skirts worn even in the drink.) Swimsuits today aren't as bulky. They're also pretty high-tech, since the predominant fabrics are man-made. Polyester, polyurethane, and, occasionally, nylon are popular fabric choices because they're durable, withstand sunlight, and repel water excellently.

Trying to keep up with the latest in beach fashions can make your head swim. So don't bother. Here are some tips to keep you in style whenever you hit the surf.

Be a boxer, guy. "It's hard to go wrong with boxer-style trunks. Boxers are flattering to everybody," says Ken Karpinski of Sterling, Virginia, image consultant to Fortune 500 companies, the U.S. military, and many corporate executives, and author of *Red Socks Don't Work*.

Boxers range from standard straight-cut, mid-thigh shorts to tapered Bermudas to the more contemporary, long, baggy look. Setting the extremes for swimsuits are the barely-there Speedos and the full-length "surfer jam" pants. "Jams are for the younger set or the trendy eccentrics," Karpinski says. "Otherwise, older men in jams look silly."

Top it off. The most flattering complement to a nice swimsuit is equally nice musculature. Barring that, anything goes: tank tops, T-shirts, or, more formally, a pullover golf shirt. It's nice if your shirt and suit match, but who cares if you're taking your top off?

Avoid sun sets. In case it's a question, forget the "cabana-style" swimsuit/shirt sets. "That's as aging as you can get. A young or middle-age man

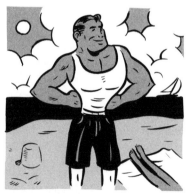

wearing a matching suit and shirt set won't look very appealing to anyone under 60," Karpinski says.

Don't go down the tubes. For fashionable footwear, stick with sandals, flip-flops, or sneakers—with or without short tennis socks. Never wear tube socks on the beach.

Don't play yacht, see. The old-style yachting look has sunk. Thurston Howell III from *Gilligan's Island* was the only person who ever looked right wearing white pants, double-breasted navy blazer with gold buttons, and an ascot. The only acceptable time for this antiquated image is if you're rich enough to afford a yacht the size of Rhode Island.

Get wet. There's a reason why some magazine cover models are repeatedly shown with their hair slicked back and perspiration beading down their bodies. It's because the wet look is sexy. Whether you're wet from water or sweat, a sleek, moist physique is an attractive one. Make the most of this at the beach by getting wet early. Slick back your hair and don your sunglasses. Adding a little lemon juice to your hair will keep it wet-looking and will help lighten it, giving you an ersatz beach-bum look when you hit dry dock later.

Lighten up already. Who gets noticed at the beach? Okay, besides beautiful women in skimpy suits. It's children. Why? Because kids play at the beach. They have fun. They run, dig, bury, scream, chase, and, yes, swim. Take a tip from the tots and do the same. Having fun chasing your kid, building sand castles, or belly-busting waves shows the world that you're confident, approachable, and easygoing. So while the other men are too concerned with looking cool or stoic, unabashedly express your own joie de vivre. You'll have more fun and look better at the same time.

Stop staring. Classy guys don't ogle.

Should You Wear Speedos? A Self-Test

Stroll down the talcum powder coast of any pristine beach and eventually you'll come across a chalky, quivering mass of flesh that has washed up on shore. It's jellylike, but no jellyfish. It's a fat guy in Speedos, those sleek, chic, Olympic-style, bikini-brief swimsuits made from as much material as a baby wipe.

Speedos aren't for everybody. Or every body, says image consultant Ken Karpinski. "A lot of men wearing Speedos are guys who swam competitively in high school or college, or they're guys who used to be really built," he says. "They think that this gives them license to wear these suits now regardless of what they look like."

Speedos make you no more a swimmer than a Dallas Cowboys jersey makes you Troy Aikman. So, for men who have a problem separating fat from fiction, Karpinski offers this simple rule of thumb: "If you have Speedos in the drawer and want to wear them, put them on when you're alone first," he says. "Then look in a full-length mirror and ask yourself, honestly, 'Would I want my young child to see this man on the beach?' "

Stylish men don't stare. If you're going to take in the sights at the beach, be discreet.

Remember your mission. Wooden takes the most refreshing and, perhaps, healthiest attitude that we've heard concerning what to wear when sunning and funning. "My wife, for example, is a personal trainer with a fabulous body, yet she wears ultra-conservative swimsuits," Wooden says. "Meanwhile, women 80 pounds overweight and pasty white are wearing the tiniest suits that you've ever seen.

"The moral of the story is, it's best to have healthy self-esteem. Wear whatever you feel comfortable in and concentrate on having a good time."

At the Restaurant

Serving Up Your Own Style

Sit up straight. Elbows off the table. Don't slurp your soup. Chew your food. Don't talk with your mouth full. Wipe your chin.

Now that you're grown up, no one cares how you eat. You can lean over the sink in your underwear, strap on a feed bag, and whoop it up. But while she was at it all those years ago, your mother should have told you *why* table manners were so important. Because she didn't, we will. People—often, people important to you—judge you by how you handle yourself at a meal.

"How you come across in a restaurant, your manners, the way that you deal with people—in short, how you act in this type of atmosphere says more about you than almost anything else can," says Jeff Livingston, Ph.D., past director of the National Association of Business Consultants in Raleigh, North Carolina, and an information analyst for Cisco Systems in Research Triangle Park, North Carolina.

Home away from Home

American men eat out a lot—an average of 4.3 times per week. The more money we make, the more often we eat out. Many of these meals are business-related. "Knowing what's expected in a restaurant is just as important as knowing what's expected in a boardroom, especially considering how often we eat out," says Caitlin Storhaug, spokeswoman for the National

Restaurant Association in Washington, D.C.

"If you were taking someone to a football game, you'd be relaxed and knowledgeable, but with wining and dining it's not the same. We're in need of brushing up on restaurant knowledge," adds Jay Solomon, a chef and cooking instructor in Ithaca, New York, and author of *Seven Pillars of Health* and *Great Bowls of Fire.*

Here's how to look and act the consummate gastronome next time you're eating out, be it a business lunch or a romantic dinner.

Hunger for knowledge. If you learned everything you know about food and dining at your mother's table, it's time to grow up. There is a vast world of cuisines, each with unique tastes and unique rules of etiquette. A man of style is comfortable in all food settings. So read food magazines, go to new restaurants—especially all the ethnic food hot spots in town—and ask tons of questions.

"You don't need a culinary arts degree, but it looks more perceptive of you if you know what you're talking about. It plays a role in the image you're projecting," Solomon says.

Be kind to the help. "The way you deal with waiters and the staff says a lot about how you deal with people in general," Livingston says. Be polite and professional, not condescending or overbearing. Also, understand that there is an art and science to waiting a table properly. A good waiter observes how the meal is progressing from a distance and silently, effi-

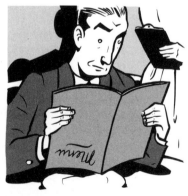

ciently, takes care of your needs, be it providing an extra knife, removing dishes, refilling water glasses, or presenting the check.

Follow basic etiquette. You should know all this, but here goes.

• Keep good posture. No slouching in your seat.

• Say "please" and "thank you" always.

• Your napkin is not a bib. Keep it on your lap, unless you're wiping your mouth between bites. Leave it on your chair when you go to the bathroom, and folded on your plate when you leave.

- Cut your meat one bite at a time.
- Keep your elbows off the table while eating; you may lightly rest them there between courses.
- Don't talk with your mouth full.
- Don't add anything to your food until you've tasted it.
- Don't pig out, particularly at a business meal. You're not eating to fill up; you're still in a meeting, remember.

Launch a stealth question. Want more information but are afraid to ask? Disguise your question. You'll look erudite. "I don't think that men in general ask enough questions of the wait staff. It's almost as if we're afraid of showing our vulnerability," Solomon says. "Disguise your question by saying something like, 'Could you elaborate on precisely how your steak tartare is prepared?'"

Follow the waiter's lead. Meals are inherently organized, so they make swell agendas for your mealtime discussions. Start with appetizers and drinks. This equals chitchat and small talk. It's the getting-to-know-you phase of the conversation. Then comes the entrée—and the meat of your discussion. It's the longest part of the meal and meant for the most important conversation. Finally, dessert and coffee, if your guest is so inclined, which is when you wrap up loose ends and revert to chitchat for nice closure.

Admit your ignorance. Having trouble with the menu? Don't fake it, advises former chef Aliza Green of Elkins Park, Pennsylvania, a culinary consultant, food columnist for the *Philadelphia Daily News*, and author of *Georges Perrier's Le Bec-Fin Cookbook.* Ask the waiter how to pronounce words, how dishes are prepared, and whether your choices go well together. Remember that intelligent questions make you seem intelligent.

"Believe me, it's better to be up front and ask than to pretend and order the 'soup doo-jow-er,'" Green says. "Menu problems are common in ethnic restaurants and fancy French and Italian restaurants, but the staff is trained to answer questions. It beats not knowing what you've ordered and being disappointed or surprised when the food comes."

Choose easy foods. If you are discussing business or trying to impress new people over a meal, pick foods that are easy to manage with a fork or spoon or that are easily cut into bite-size pieces. When conducting business, avoid sandwiches, hot wings, and any other food you eat with your hands. Even salads can be hard to handle if the greens aren't shredded to small pieces. Good choices include boneless chicken breasts, fish (but not shellfish), pasta dishes (but be careful not to slurp or you'll get oil or marinara on your shirt), and soups (same warning).

Wine—don't whine. "Wines are probably the most difficult and intimidating thing to order because nobody really knows much about them," Green says. "Instead, give your server or wine steward guidelines and ask for suggestions."

Vino parameters include how much you're willing to spend ($30 to $50 a bottle is a good mid-range), preferences (white or red, heavy or light, strong or fruity), and something that will go with your meal (fish, veal, beef, vegetarian).

Gracefully handle poor service. If your service is in need of a tune-up, discreetly excuse yourself mid-meal and ask to speak to the manager. Then politely have your say. Don't wait until you're done eating and your outing is ruined. And never argue, be rude, or condescend.

Pay with panache. Don't get into an "I'll-pay-no-let-me-pay" debate. Typically, in business situations, the instigator of the meeting picks up the tab. If the protocol is unclear, it is best to determine who will pay *prior* to the meal. If you end up getting treated, remember to offer thanks. If you pay, show class in handling the payment by doing it discreetly and swiftly, calculating the tip silently in your head.

For a Photograph

Looking Good's a Snap

There, permanently immortalized on emulsion and glossy paper is a ruthless reminder of your awkward adolescence: your high school yearbook picture.

As if acne, first dates, and a changing voice weren't enough.

Unfortunately, embarrassing photos don't end there. Life is an endless stream of Kodak moments, and every picture of you fixes forever who you were at that point in time. Wedding pictures. Birthday pictures. Holiday pictures. Reunion pictures. That embarrassing potty training photo that your mother showed every serious date you brought home.

"The scary part is that people judge books by their covers: How you look in a picture is the way that people perceive you," says Sam Doerfler, the booking agent for male models at the well-known Ford modeling agency in New York City.

How to Shine for a Shutterbug

You don't have to look like Robert Redford or Denzel Washington to look good on film. The experts say that everyone's photogenic. The trick is to treat a photo shoot like you would an important business meeting: Prepare in advance, and have a clear picture in your mind of what you hope to get out of it.

Here's how to improve your image and boost your style by coming out picture-perfect every time.

Now then, say cheese.

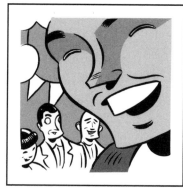

Take a practice roll. Ask a friend—or use a tripod and timer—to take pictures of yourself while you experiment with your facial expressions and poses, suggests David Wolfe of The Doneger Group.

"Most people look ill at ease before a camera because they're not sure what the camera sees," Wolfe says. "If you practice on your own by having a lot of pictures taken of you, you won't feel so awkward.

"I'm not the most photogenic guy in the world, but I've experimented and found that when I smile real hard, it gives my face structure," he says. "When someone's ready to snap a picture, I just smile real hard and everybody says that I look great."

Check the mirror. If you're reluctant to blow $15 on a roll of film and processing, practice in front of a mirror. Just be sure to close the bathroom door so that no one worries about your sanity.

Do a background search. Before facing forward to say cheese, turn around and scan the background. Many amateur shutterbugs and an occasional pro neglect to pay enough attention to the background. That's why you sometimes appear in pictures with a tree branch, smokestack, or lamppost sticking out of your head. Make sure that the background is unobtrusive and won't make you look bad.

Take charge. If you're having your picture taken for business, say, a publicity photo for the press, talk to the photographer before the shutter starts clicking. Remember that you're the subject, and if you hired the photographer, you're also the customer. Describe what you want the picture to convey. What you want it to say about you. The mood you want to create. What the picture will be used for and where it will appear.

"And always ask to see

the photographer's portfolio," recommends Doerfler. "That tells you a lot about his skill and talent. If you don't like what you see, you're better off finding someone else for your shoot."

Trust the pros. Yes, if you've hired the photographer, then you're the boss. But that said, he's the expert. Outside of setting the framework for what you want your photo to accomplish and giving your opinion on what you think works best for you in way of lighting, poses, and backgrounds, step aside and let the pros do their job. Constantly second-guessing the expert will make you look insecure or vain.

Posture for the camera. Make sure that you're not slouching. Most of us do this unconsciously because we've developed poor posture habits, or because we're really afraid of looking bad on film, so we shrink away when we should be proudly striking a pose.

Look dreamy. Gunning for that dreamy, debonair look? Here's what male models do. "Look at the lens but pretend that you're looking at something in the distance," Doerfler says. "This gives you a deep, penetrating stare and accentuates your eyes."

Turn pro. Just because we knew that you were wondering but would never ask, here's what it takes, on average, to be a professional male model.

- Height: six feet to six feet two inches; weight: 175 pounds
- Prominent cheekbones; well-defined jaw; prominent, preferably light-colored, eyes
- Good, solid build with broad shoulders and, usually, a size 40 regular jacket

Looking Good on TV

Being on TV looks easy—until you do it the first time. Only then is it possible to muster a modicum of respect for Geraldo, if only because he handles the small screen with such panache.

"TV can be difficult because there are some standards of style for TV that aren't the same as normal dress protocol," says Michael R. Losey, president and chief executive officer of the Society for Human Resource Management, a professional organization in Alexandria, Virginia. For example, while a white shirt may be okay in almost every business setting, you wouldn't wear one on TV. It will wash out your face and make you look heavier.

Here are some other things to keep in mind when the studio lights come on.

Test patterns. Don't wear white, red, or black; very thin, close stripes; horizontal stripes; or busy patterns. Each affects video quality, making you look heavier, smaller, or fuzzier on-screen, Losey says. Avoid shiny jewelry or eyeglasses, which can reflect light and wreak havoc by causing glare.

Be conservative. Wear conservative, medium-colored suits, with a light blue shirt and conservative tie. Wear bold stripes or fine stripes spaced far apart. Ask what color the studio set is and choose a contrasting color so that you don't blend in like chameleon man.

Get powdered. Always request makeup to cover unflattering blemishes that a close-up might yield. Always powder to eliminate the shine from an oily forehead or nose, Losey says.

- A 40- to 42-inch chest, 15- to 15½-inch neck, and a 33- to 34-inch sleeve
- A 32-inch waist, with 10-inch rise

At a Job Interview

Employing Style at Work

Short of an IRS audit, sitting down for a job interview is probably the most uncomfortable tête-à-tête in your adult life. Seldom are you judged so harshly, so superficially, and so quickly for something so important.

"And it's all done really before you know it," says Michael R. Losey of the Society for Human Resource Management. "The first impression that you make is the most important, and you'll be judged on it within the first two minutes."

The rest of the interview—the questions and answers, the perfunctory lunch, the building tour—are just sneaky ways for you to slip up. It's the interviewer's time to hone his opinion. And it's a time when your image, style, and good behavior should be among your most valuable assets.

The Two-Minute Drill

Those mighty two minutes of introduction mean a lot, but they're no cause for alarm. While there are a million factors you can't control in a job interview—like whether the interviewer is waiting to interview an old fraternity brother next—there are lots of things that you *can* control. Important things. Things that work to your advantage.

"The number one thing that you're evaluated on the moment you walk through the door is your dress," Losey says.

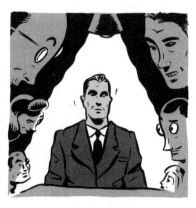

"After that, it's your general appearance, with emphasis on two characteristics: your height, weight, and their proportion, and your general overall appearance."

The average American man is five feet nine inches tall and 162 pounds. The average American executive is a little taller and a little heavier, Losey says. "Look at any chief executive officer. They're proportionally taller than average and Rock Hudson types," he says. "I've seen many occasions where people who don't fit that image are dismissed prematurely, which is sad, because leaders come in all shapes and sizes."

While you can't do much to change your height, there are lots of other strategies to adopt. And, like Losey and other experts say, what you wear is the most important starting point.

"Your clothes are your tools. They're going to set the tone for your entire interview," says image consultant Louise Elerding, president of the Association of Image Consultants International and owner of The Color Studio in Glendale, California.

Here's how to maximize your chance of landing that job by maximizing your style— clothing and all.

Dress right. This means traditional, conventional, and conservative. John T. Molloy, the nationally renowned image expert, syndicated columnist, and author of the best-selling *John T. Molloy's New Dress for Success*, suggests this lineup: a very conservative dark blue suit for the first interview; a conservative solid gray for the second; and a dark gray or dark blue pinstripe with matching vest for the grand finale meeting with the big cheese.

Your shirt is always white, well-pressed, and starched, Molloy says; your tie is conservative, with a small pattern that doesn't reek of Ivy League.

Be a single guy. Avoid double-breasted suits because

they lend an air that's too powerful for an interview. You want your suit to say conservative, corporate, approachable, and friendly. Not showman or emcee.

Do your homework. You're an intelligent, competent, and capable guy, and you want that to come across in the interview. Nothing boosts your image (and confidence) as much as being well-informed. Kate Wendleton, in her book *Through the Brick Wall*, offers these tips.

- Do library research on the company. Know what it has been doing in the industry, what its long-term goals are, and what its financial standing is.
- Call the company's public relations department for a media kit and annual report.
- Ask others in the industry about the company.
- Show up early and read the company literature in the reception area.
- Talk with people in the lobby, including receptionists and secretaries. Be a people watcher.

Bring a cue card. Wendleton also suggests boiling down everything you want to cover onto a three- by five-inch index card that addresses why the employer should hire you; a summary of yourself, your credentials, personality, and what you have to offer; two key accomplishments that support your interest in the position; a counterargument to the employer's most likely objection to you, if any; and why you want to work specifically for this company.

Knowing this and rehearsing your "pitch" beforehand makes you look polished. The beauty of an index card is that you can carry it in your pocket and review it while waiting.

Follow JFK's advice. Don't be self-centered; it's an easy pitfall. To paraphrase the late President John F. Kennedy's inaugural address, ask not what the company can do for

The First Time

The first real job interview after school is nerve-racking. Since you're still living with milk-crate furniture—and now student loans—you can't afford a professional wardrobe to brag about. Here's how the entry-level guy can achieve maximum style with minimal money.

Ban the beard. Until you've "arrived" in your career and can call the shots a little more liberally, conform to what's expected: clean-shaven.

Buy the blazer. If you can't afford a suit, buy a dark blue blazer. If you have one left over from your fraternity days, make sure that it's a classic design and free of beer stains and cigarette burns. Pair a blue blazer with khaki pants, a white shirt and a silk tie, and you have a respectable entry-level interview outfit.

Dandy your dogs. Don't neglect your feet, or, more specifically, your socks and shoes. "Shoes and socks are something that an interviewer is bound to see as you cross your legs," says Princess Jenkins of Majestic Images International. "Make sure that your shoes are shined and your socks patterned, matching, and of the same color."

you. Ask what you can do for the company.

Send your regards. Image consultant and makeup artist Princess Jenkins, owner of Majestic Images International, an image consulting firm in New York City, says that a thank-you card is the gold standard of professional and personal etiquette.

"It's a tiny step, but if you're interviewing against five people and you're the only one who sends a follow-up, it could be the edge that you need," says Jenkins, who also teaches professional image and job-hunting skills to community service organizations. "How quickly you send a handwritten thank-you shows your manners and the kind of person that you are."

On Casual Friday

Dressing Down with Style

Workers may love Casual Friday, but some fashion experts fear that it may signal the decline of style in the workplace.

"Thanks to Casual Friday, corporate dress has really become a problem. We've become a nation of slobs," frets fashion expert Leon Hall of New York City, who is creative director for International Apparel Mart in Dallas, spokesperson for The Fashion Association, and a frequent fashion commentator and trend forecaster. "People say that Casual Friday is a new way of dressing, but it isn't license for sloppiness and slovenliness, and that's what has happened."

While other experts aren't so emphatic—particularly casual wear manufacturers—it's clear that Casual Friday has changed the rules about what's appropriate to wear to work. And if you want to be Joe Friday, you need to understand what the new style standards are.

A Casual Acquaintance

In many offices, Casual Friday got its sneakered foot in the door via local charities, such as the United Way and United Cerebral Palsy. These organizations in the late 1980s and early 1990s found that employees were eager to pledge money if it meant that they could dress casually at work.

Pittsburgh-based ALCOA, the world's largest aluminum manufacturer, for example, went totally casual in September 1991

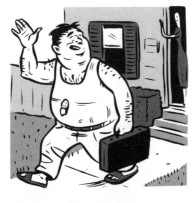

following a United Way campaign. Managers permitted employees who pledged early to the United Way to dress casually for the remainder of the fund-raising campaign. Response was so overwhelming—and productivity and morale so noticeably improved—that the company made casual dress a permanent policy.

"Casual dress can have clear advantages, at virtually no cost, for most corporations and industries," says Michael R. Losey of the Society for Human Resource Management.

Yet, as Losey points out, Casual Friday has caused considerable consternation, too. "Just because you're dressing casually doesn't mean that there aren't standards. In many cases, the corporate casual concept has just muddied the standards," he says.

Hall says that he knows of some companies in New York City that are so fed up with conflicting definitions of casual that they've adopted Dress-Up Friday to restore some sense of fashion order.

Losey's organization, along with Levi Strauss and Company, looked into Casual Friday by surveying 505 human resource managers nationwide in 1996. They found that:

- 90 percent of the companies allowed workers to wear casual clothing at least some of the time, which was up 27 percent from 1992
- 42 percent of the companies allow casual clothing once a week; 33 percent permit it daily
- 63 percent of all companies had a written dress policy regarding casual dress

What is the bottom line for bosses? Casual dress improves morale, is perceived as an employee benefit, saves employees money, and attracts new workers, the survey says.

According to the Society for Human Resource Management/Levi Strauss and Company survey, here's what most men wear on a designated casual day at work.

- Polo shirts, short-sleeve shirts
- Casual slacks, jeans
- Leather shoes

As a general guide, that's a pretty safe standard for a dress-down day. But does that make it the official uniform for Casual Friday? Not necessarily. Here are some tips to help you make sense of the new office anarchy.

Watch the boss. What might cut it at XYZ Advertising Agency probably won't make it past the security guard at IBM. What's appropriate varies from city to city, region to region, company to company.

"Your office might be more conservative," says Hall. "The easiest thing to do is to look around and see what the bosses are wearing. If they're not wearing sneakers, neither should you."

Tee off. T-shirts most often are a no-no on casual day, so think twice, even if your company allows them. If you opt for a T-shirt, make it plain and solid-colored, perhaps with a single breast pocket. And it doesn't matter whether your musical tastes run toward Sinatra or the Sex Pistols. Save the concert T-shirts for the weekend.

Be a trailblazer. You'll never go wrong with a blazer or sport coat. They jazz up even the most casual outfits, including jeans. And if it's too dressy, you can always take it off. "Corporate casual revolves around the sport coat. Along with a coordinating shirt and trousers, it's a definite cornerstone to a corporate casual wardrobe," says Marvin Pieland, manager and clothing consultant for Saks Fifth Avenue Club for Men in New York City.

Select a shirt. Safe shirts for casual wear include collared polo shirts, solid colors or muted prints, banded-collar shirts, denim shirts, neatly pressed oxford button-downs, and stylish rugby shirts. Stick with chambray, denim, or flannel for a softer look than standard starched cotton.

Life after Friday

Everybody's talking about what to wear on Casual Friday, but no one—until now—has ever addressed the second-most important casual dress question in America: What do you wear on Working Saturday?

Blessed are the few who can work a full month without at least a quick stop by the office on a Saturday morning. Even if you're finishing up that million-dollar sales proposal, few things could more seriously sidetrack your rise to the corner office than having the boss see you in your shredded jeans and "Take this job and shove it" T-shirt. Sure, you're in the office on your own time. But remember that you are in the office.

"You have to be sensitive to your image any time you're somewhere where you can meet someone in a professional sense," warns Marvin Pieland of Saks Fifth Avenue Club for Men. "Remember that it's not always so much whether you're comfortable but whether people will be comfortable looking at you.

"When people see you in a ratty T-shirt and cutoffs, it shakes their perception of you if your image is otherwise conservative, stylish, and inspiring," Pieland says.

Don't wear something that's going to say or imply something negative about you or your credibility.

Pick the right pants. You can't go wrong with dress slacks, khakis, or chinos. Even a nice pair of jeans *might* be okay, as long as they're not the kind you'd wear horseback riding and as long as they're dressed up with an oxford shirt and blazer.

Err on the side of fashion. If you're not sure what goes in your office, dress up more than you need to. "It's safer to dress up. You can always dress down—remove your jacket, roll up your sleeves, and loosen your tie. You can't go the other way," says image consultant Ken Karpinski.

At a Business Meeting

Getting Your Point Across

Business meetings are important. They prove how many managers your company can get along without.

Okay, meetings are a little more important than that. While it's certainly true that some companies hold far too many meetings that drag on for far too long, you need to realize that the impression that you make in those settings will go a long way toward determining how high you climb on the corporate ladder.

"How you handle yourself at an important meeting says a lot about your style and personality, and most of what it boils down to is this: Are you conducting yourself appropriately?" says Michael R. Losey of the Society for Human Resource Management.

"In other words, are you honest, straightforward, and credible? Are you showing that you're bright, informed, and balanced in your decision making?" Losey asks. "It's the absence of these elements at a meeting that gives people the impression that you have poor style."

The Secret Meaning of Meetings

We tried to research how many minutes the average American spends in meetings, but we ran into a bit of trouble. So we called a meeting. In mid-session, we formed a committee, which, in turn, created four sub-committees to continue the research. After most of our dead-line passed, nothing had

improved, so we tabled our research for now.

Sound familiar?

Determining how much time Americans spend in meetings truly is difficult. According to Winston Fletcher in his book *Meetings, Meetings*, the average executive spends 3½ hours a week in formal committee meetings, and another full day in informal conferences and consultations. One British survey, Fletcher says, found that our U.K. brethren spend fully half their time in formal and informal discussions. Not surprisingly, the higher up on the corporate totem pole you are, the more likely you are to be in a meeting. Moreover, estimates suggest that just 1 meeting in 10 is productive.

Nevertheless, unless you're unemployed or very unambitious at work, you will be spending a lot of time in meetings, so make the most of them.

"Important meetings shouldn't be your training ground. Make sure that you know what to do and how to do it before you're addressing peers, clients, co-workers, or the boss," advises Hendrie Weisinger, Ph.D., a psychologist, business consultant, and author of *Anger at Work*, *Nobody's Perfect*, and *Dr. Weisinger's Anger Work-Out Book*.

Your Personal Agenda

If you want to make a strong impression, you have to have a clear picture of what it is that you want to accomplish.

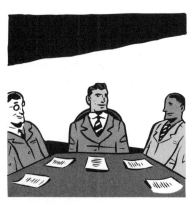

"Remember that everyone has their own agenda in a meeting, and how well you're prepared—in dress, demeanor, information, body English—helps get your agenda passed," says Dr. Jeff Livingston of Cisco Systems.

Here's what you need to know to look good and make a positive impression at meetings.

Know the subject. One of the reasons that most

meetings are unproductive is the failure to focus on the topic. And part of that can be pinned on people unfamiliar with the subject going off on tangents. Find out what's on the agenda (get an advanced copy if at all possible) and then do your homework. Dig out any reports or background information relating to it and review them beforehand. It may make perfect sense, based on current information, to make a case for the company moving into widget production. But you're not going to come off well if you don't know that, 10 years ago, the company marketed a line of widgets—and almost went bankrupt because of it.

Know the players. Football coaches review films of their opponents before playing the game. You should do the same thing, if only mentally. Find out who will be at the meeting and prep yourself on their individual styles and opinions. Know who's likely to be an ally and who's likely to be an opponent. Then figure out the neutral parties—and make a point of speaking to them before the meeting.

Avoid speech making. A bad meeting is like a session of Congress—a series of disjointed speeches that represent the "little people back in my department" that no one listens to and takes everyone nowhere fast. Leave your soapbox behind; never rant and rave at a meeting.

Make your point fast, then elaborate as needed. Typically, listeners start to tune out just 10 seconds after a person starts to speak. To capture people's attention and interest, state your point immediately and then elaborate. Never start a comment with "I was thinking on my way in this morning" or some such useless verbiage. Rather, say, "I think that we should consider splitting the two departments. Here's why."

Schmooze. Show up a couple of minutes early and chitchat to establish good rapport and grease the social wheels. The worst thing that you can do is walk in late. You might as well hang a sign around your neck that says "Unprepared."

Try a little levity. Some well-placed, appropriate humor and enthusiasm go a long way. "Anyone with the resilience to stay perky (in meetings) will frequently be able to put one over on the other participants when they are comatose or even asleep," Fletcher advises.

Play by the rules. More companies are adopting unusual meeting formats and structures, often taught by outside consultants who specialize in creative problem solving and meeting management. Some of these new methods can be pretty weird. Nonetheless, don't resist these new approaches, even if they force you to do an occasionally silly thing. It's an insult to your boss to be a negative force or a drag on the proceedings, particularly when he spent good money hiring an outside facilitator. In public, always support new approaches. If you think that it was an absurd exercise, deal with that *after* the meeting and in private.

Be positive, not negative. Sometimes, it's the easiest thing to do: cut down other's ideas, find the flaws in a plan, question the wisdom of a policy. You learned this with your first set of building blocks: It's easier to destroy things than to build them. But men of style know that there is far greater reward and pleasure in being a positive force for change. If you don't like it, don't just criticize it; offer alternative—and smarter—solutions.

Convey charisma. We've all dealt with someone who came across as unnecessarily crass and condescending. Didn't do much for his image, and it won't do much for yours. Strive to show empathy, compassion, enthusiasm, and affability. In short, exude charisma.

"Charisma is coming off as charming and friendly, like you really care. I've found that this isn't something you're born with or learn, it's something you evolve into," Dr. Weisinger says. "It's a by-product of your experiences and personal effort. No one sits down and teaches you charisma."

That's not to say you should be a rollover guy. Just come congenially; let them see your inner iron only when you need to.

Playing Sports
Know How to Dress Like a Pro

It's no surprise that sports profoundly influence style. The shirts and shorts that athletes wear and endorse have become the accoutrements of choice for many. But that's not the only way image factors into sports. Regardless of *whose* product you're wearing, *what* you're wearing matters even more, says image consultant Ken Karpinski.

"Endorsements aside, the clothing conventions in sports matter because people expect to see certain things in certain sports," Karpinski says. "People expect golfers to dress in a particular way. They expect tennis players to wear a particular outfit. By honoring those conventions, you're giving yourself instant credibility. It's almost as if you're saying, simply by what you're wearing, that you know the game and you know the rules."

Case in point: You may be a scratch golfer, but if you try hitting the greens at an upscale golf course in tattered cutoff jeans and a tie-dyed T-shirt, you won't get past the surly starter. But if you're dressed appropriately, "you'll probably find that people are more forgiving and accepting, even if you're not particularly skillful," Karpinski says.

Basic Training

Here are the basics of dressing right—and acting right—on the course, court, track, and even in the backwoods.

Golf

Robert Tyre Jones, an up-and-coming American golfer in the 1920s, established himself as a fashion maven on the greens

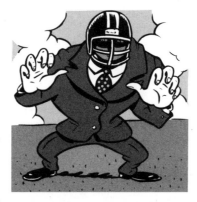

by popularizing golf's ugliest creation: the two-tone saddle shoe.

Originally created by Spalding in 1906 for tennis and squash players, the saddle shoe never caught on. After marketing them to golfers, Spalding discovered an unlikely sponsor in Jones. Others followed, like the fastidious and fashionable Bobby Jones, and the saddle shoe rose to stardom.

You don't necessarily need saddle shoes to look like a pro, but here's what you will need.

Dress for success. According to David Gould, a former executive editor of *Golf Illustrated*, you don't need to wear traditional tartan knickers and a Scottish cap to look good at golf. Choose loose-fitting 100 percent cotton shirts and pants for warm-weather play. Avoid the "ugly-golfer" look by wearing solid colors in muted shades. If you need a jacket, make it a windbreaker. And opt for spikes. Even a cheap pair with leather uppers provide the right traction at a cost of about $60 a pair at a discount store.

Don't forget your balls. Always pack more than you'll need. Especially if you're playing with the big boys and don't want to be an anchor. (Playing poorly is one thing; holding up your boss is another.) Know the brand and number of your balls. Good golfers do. It looks better to say "I'm looking for a Maxfli 3" than "Uh, it was white."

Don't fake it. Working the links and climbing the corporate ladder go hand in hand. But if you're not a good golfer, or have never played, don't fake your way through a round, suggests Dr. Jeff Livingston of Cisco Systems.

"If someone invited me to play golf for a business-social, I'd do anything that I could to get out of it," Dr. Livingston says. "If I couldn't, I'd be up front and admit that I don't play very well or have never played at all. People appreciate honesty. Especially if the other guy's good, he won't appreciate you bogging down the foursome."

Tennis

Augusta Moran never made it real big in competitive tennis, but at Wimbledon's British Open in 1949 she emblazoned her name in history. Moran, an attractive 27-year-old American dubbed "Gorgeous Gussie," bounced on court wearing a scandalously short, white skirt that just barely covered lace-trimmed panties. The de rigeur outfits at the time, for men and women, were modest white shorts.

Although Moran was eliminated in her third match, the mark that she made on tennis was indelible. After a media circus of attention, lace began appearing on everything from swimsuits to ski suits. Her short skirt remains the norm for women today.

We don't suggest you take such scandalous measures with your wardrobe, but here's what we do suggest when you find yourself in court.

Dress white. "When I was playing, 95 percent of the clothing was white or very soft pastel. It wasn't unusual for a club not to let you on a court if you weren't wearing white," says Karpinski, who used to play and teach tennis for a living and who owned several pro shops.

"Most every sport has opened up to what's allowable, but you can never go wrong in the tried and true. In fact, they might even think that you're a good player because of it," he says.

Consider simply wearing a plain cotton T-shirt or polo shirt, comfortable nylon shorts, mid-priced tennis shoes, and white socks. Be appropriate—no jean cutoffs or raggy T-shirts.

Be twinkle-toes. Tennis isn't about just hitting a ball. It's about moving. You have to be in position before you can return a volley, no? Stay on the balls of your feet for short, fast steps. Think lightfooted. Not cement shoes.

A Sporting Chance

The softball field or local walking track is more than just a proving ground for your athletic prowess. It's a chance to network and refine your social skills. That's what a national Bozell Worldwide/U.S. News survey says.

Almost 90 percent of all sports participants surveyed think that sports help teach people to get along with others, especially people of different ethnic and racial backgrounds. Seventy percent of those polled also said that sports helped them deal with the opposite sex better.

Despite theories to the contrary, the survey found that most Americans (71 percent) rejected the idea that sports promote violent behavior, and 70 percent agreed that athletes deserve every bit of respect and fame they get in U.S. culture.

So when it comes to presenting your maximum style, sports might be just the ticket to rounding out the physical and interpersonal sides of your image all at once.

Even if it doesn't improve the accuracy of your shots, you'll get a better workout and appear more graceful.

Make a racket. Look like a seasoned pro by holding your racket like one. Beginners almost always heft their rackets around by the handle. It's not a hatchet. It's a tool. And an expensive one at that. Hold your racket by cradling it in your non-hitting hand, just below the head.

Cycling

Cycling is a great sport when it comes to image. Few sports offer such a wide array of cool gear and awesome exercise. Sunglasses. Spandex shorts. Helmets. Little rearview mirrors that clip on to your helmets. Oh, yeah, and the bikes. On the physical side, there's aerobic conditioning, muscle building, wind sprints, distance rides, and outdoor adventures on mountain bikes.

Most important, though, "cyclists are buff. They have streamlined bodies and powerful thighs and calves that look like they're made of titanium," says Lisa Gosselin, executive editor of *Bicycling* magazine.

Along with all these opportunities to look good come opportunities to look foolish. To avoid that, consider these tips.

Wear clothes made for biking. Part of cycling means suiting up for a ride. That means wearing cycling shorts, jersey, socks, and shoes.

"T-shirts and shorts don't cut it any more," Gosselin says. Why? Because cycling clothes are not only more stylish but also far more pragmatic. Cycling shorts have padded crotches to prevent chafing. Jerseys are brightly colored to keep you visible, plus they have handy pockets sewn into the back. ("Watch how fast something falls out of a front pocket," Gosselin says.) Socks are ankle-height so that they don't get stuck in a gear, and shoes should be cycling shoes because they have extra-stiff soles for support.

"The telltale sign of a bike schmo is sneakers. Worse yet, sneakers and high socks," Gosselin says. Spring for clip-on cycling shoes. They're best for form and power, "and they look pro."

The problem with cycling clothing is that it is often garish, filled with screaming colors and huge company logos. This isn't you? No problem. You can get biking shorts in straight-black Lycra, or you can buy touring shorts that look more like ordinary shorts but are made for long-distance riding. Slightly muted shirts are available as well to make you conspicuous enough to not get run over by a car but modest enough not to get mistaken for a billboard.

Use your head. But not to break your fall. Statistics show that 27 percent of all bicyclists own or have use of a helmet, yet

The Long and Short of Shorts

Only a decade ago, your choice of athletic shorts was pretty much limited to short, tight basketball shorts. The kind you wore in gym class. The only other option, not suitable for athletics, was the longish, casual Bermuda shorts.

Things aren't so clear now. Shorts come in all shapes and sizes, and you're no longer limited by cotton. Spandex, cotton, neoprene, and polyester blends are the norm, and short lengths are rising and lowering like the tide of women's hemlines.

"It seemed pretty clear with spandex. Just five years ago, it looked like guys were wearing tight, mini scuba gear," says Princess Jenkins of Majestic Images International. "Now you have Michael Jordan wearing basketball shorts with his crotch down around his knees."

As far as which direction you should be heading in, Jenkins and other experts suggest wearing whatever you

three-quarters rarely or never use it. Just 13 percent of riders always or almost always use a helmet.

Consider this: The only thing dorkier than an ugly or ill-fitting helmet is an open head wound and brain damage.

"If you haven't bought a helmet in years, you have many to choose from. They're sleek, colorful, and have as many as 24 air vents, which means that they're light, cool, and good-looking," Gosselin says. "Make sure that your helmet fits squarely on your noggin and that the chin strap is taut, not tight."

Other protective gear that you need includes gloves, or your hands will look like chopped meat on your first fall, and sunglasses. Not only will you look sleeker in shades but also they'll keep bugs out of your eyes.

Breathe easy. Minding your breathing keeps your body oxygenated. It also keeps you from panting like a dog when you're done.

feel most comfortable in. "And whatever works best for your body shape, height, and weight," she says. "The reality is that, in terms of activewear, trends change; so you can either try to be on top of the latest fashion or just be more practical about it."

One thing that you might want to consider is wearing neoprene shorts. A study of 44 rugby players found that those who wore neoprene shorts agitated old hamstring injuries less frequently. The reason is that neoprene has excellent thermal retention, meaning that it keeps your muscles warmer than, say, cotton. This is especially vital to the hamstring, which is a common sports injury and the muscle most frequently injured in the thigh. Just don't rely on your shorts to keep your legs shipshape. When it comes to preventing injury, nothing takes the place of proper warm-ups, stretching, and cooldowns.

you look like you're armed for combat. A lot of people skip it, especially in beach cities where it's fashionable to skate the boardwalk.

Here's what you need to succeed at in-line skating.

Don't spare the pads. You *knew* we'd say this. Consider that experienced skaters can go as fast as 17 miles per hour. Consider also that in-line skating injuries, as a rule, tend to rank "more severe" than roller skating or skateboarding. In 1994 alone, 75,000 trips were made to the emergency room for in-line skating injuries, a quarter of which were for wrist injuries. Pads don't look goofy. Road rash and protruding fractures look goofy.

Pamper your hands. If you insist on not wearing gear, ignore the wrist guards. Fracture studies at Thomas Jefferson University Hospital in Philadelphia found that in-line skating wrist guards protect you more from road rash than from fractures. So you might as well wear a set of less-expensive leather cycling gloves if you want.

Wear a helmet. Although only 4.8 percent of in-line skating injuries occur to the head, compared to 11.8 percent for cyclists, anytime you mess with the head, you run the chance of long-term or disabling damage.

Show style with your skates off. What's the point of looking buff with your skates on if you look like a dork in white tube socks and shorts after you take them off? Consider Wigwam's In-Line Skate Sock. It's a long athletic sock made from synthetic fibers especially for skating. It's great at wicking moisture away from your feet and has an extra padded elastic ankle panel to ensure that it stays in place while you're cruising the boardwalk.

Master the most important move. One move that trips up skaters all the time is stopping. If you want to look graceful on in-line

Your best bet is to breathe through your nose whenever you can. It warms, filters, and humidifies the air that you're taking in.

Shave legs—and time. If you're a serious rider, shave your legs. It'll show off the rock-hard quads and calves that you've earned, plus it reduces wind drag and makes cleaning road rash easier. Start with a depilatory, like Nair, and finish with a razor. Continue throughout the riding season, or your legs will have a crew cut by week's end.

In-Line Skating

In-line skating, or Rollerblading as it's often called, is the sport of the 1990s. It's one of the fastest-growing sports, having increased 51 percent to 9.4 million enthusiasts in just one year in 1992. Today, it's estimated that more than 15 million people enjoy in-line skating.

Unfortunately, in-line skating requires you to wear enough protective gear to make

skates and can only master one move, know how to stop.

Running

Running is one of the easiest sports to neglect when it comes to style and image. After all, at its lowest common denominator, you only need shorts, shoes, and two legs. But don't get caught off guard.

"While lots of runners don't necessarily look 'good' while running—President Bill Clinton is a prime example with his baggy shorts—the image of a runner is an extremely positive one," says Amby Burfoot, executive editor of *Runner's World* magazine and a former winner of the Boston Marathon. "Runners set goals. Runners are disciplined. Everyone admires people who set tough goals and finish what they start."

Here's how to run in style.

Don't sweat the sweats. Those old cotton sweatpants from gym class might have been okay for the 30-yard dash in sixth-grade, but they won't do today. You want pants made with breathable fibers that won't get bogged down with sweat. Cotton will. Options include high-tech sweats or even tights. The upside to tights and shorts made from, say, neoprene is that they tend to keep your muscles a little warmer, which prevents cramping and pulls. They also look sleeker and sexier than sweats.

As for shirts, forget T-shirts. "Runners wear polyester these days. The new polyester is as soft as cotton and much more breathable," Burfoot says. "Runners produce so much body heat and sweat that they need breathable fabrics that wick moisture away."

Finally, buy running shoes. A good pair costs $75 to $90; a great pair costs a little more. High-arch shoes are generally most cushioned; low-arch shoes are less cushioned and built for better control.

Run with pride. You hear a lot about runner's high—that mystical moment when the endorphins kick in on a long run. Then you see some guy shuffling down the road, hunched over with a tortured look on his face. Does it

look like he's having fun? A classic running style helps make a stylish runner. Keep your head up, your body erect, and your stride comfortable and graceful. Don't bounce up and down, take exaggerated steps, or slog through the motions with head bowed and eyes riveted on the ground. Your arms should swing naturally at your sides, without twisting too much in front.

Enjoy the energy. Here's something that makes running appealing to anyone: Run often and you won't run out of energy often. It's a paradox, but, as Burfoot says, "runners are noticeably more energetic people."

"It's a hard principle to grasp. You think you run so that you get tired, but the truth is that when you run, you get re-energized," Burfoot says. On the more tangible side, "runners are mostly trim. Not too skinny, but trim. You look younger and wear your clothes better and longer."

Hiking and Walking

Walking today is one of the most popular forms of exercise for men as well as women. One national study found that 9 in 10 American adults regularly walk outside their homes for one reason or another. The average person took 15 walks in the last mild-weather month, and 8 in 10 people walk to enjoy nature. A full three-quarters walk for exercise. The cities with the most walkers are Boston; Pittsburgh; Washington, D.C.; New York; and Philadelphia.

According to the Centers for Disease Control and Prevention and the American College of Sports Medicine, Americans should get at least 30 minutes of moderate-intensity exercise on most days of the week, which, according to the experts, is the equivalent of briskly walking two miles.

Here's how to walk in style, with some special advice on hiking.

If the shoe fits, wear it. If you're walking or hiking regularly, invest in footwear. You'll look every bit the part, but, more important, your image won't be hampered by unsightly blisters or limping because you sprained your ankle. Good walking shoes should have firm arches, sturdy lacing, and a strong heel. Hiking boots are another matter.

"Hiking boots are big," says Kirt Mancuso, marketing services manager for Florsheim, a footwear manufacturer in Chicago. "Agricultural footwear fashion is in. It's a cross between the gritty grunge look of Seattle and middle America."

Mancuso suggests that your hiking boots be waterproof ("just in case") and made of sturdy maintenance-free leather with tractor-like lug soles for extra traction. "Hand stitching also matters to a lot of guys who've had the experience of wearing tough-looking shoes that don't hold up well," he says.

Pass the test. As with all shoes, give your walking shoes and hiking boots the thumb test. "That's when you press your thumb on the inside sole, where your heel would go, and ask yourself if your foot will be happy there for hours on end," Mancuso says.

Wear all-weather fare. "The basic principles of sportswear are the same whether you're walking around the city or hiking out in the mountains," says David Secunda, executive director of the Outdoor Recreation Coalition of America in Boulder, Colorado. "The only difference is that it's not a matter of life or death if you get a little wet in an urban setting."

To that end, keep in mind the three elements of all outdoor activewear: wicking, the fabric's ability to move moisture away from your body; insulating; and waterproofing. If you're going to spend lots of time outdoors, insulating and waterproofing are your most important factors. If you're doing some light to moderate exercise—but won't be stranded on a mountain at dark—wicking takes priority.

Science and Sport

Sports clothing, or activewear, is a ripe field for technology. The active 1980s were a cash cow for textile manufacturers who scrambled to create the perfect clothing for the sports-minded. They paid special attention to creating clothing with these four properties: moisture wicking, water resistance, elasticity, and thermal protection.

Spandex is probably the best-known clothing creation in sportswear. It's a member of the elastomeric fibers, a man-made group of materials characterized by their ability to stretch up to 800 percent without tearing. Created first by Du Pont in 1958 under the brand name Lycra, spandex is actually made of polyurethane. It has single-handedly changed the face—or, more accurately, the legs, tummies, and buttocks—of our nation.

Other innovations in sports clothing include the widespread use of materials that trap body heat. These include Polytherm by the U.S. Department of Agriculture and Thinsulate by 3M. They're big sellers in clothing made to withstand outdoor exposure, such as hunting, camping, or hiking gear. A final innovation is Sway. Developed by Toray in 1989, Sway is coated nylon that changes color when the temperature changes. Variations change color when exposed to sunlight. Although these colorful innovations made a brief debut in the late 1980s as novelty clothing (remember Hypercolor T-shirts?), experts think that they may be more pragmatically employed to warn skiers or hikers when they've had too much exposure to the elements.

Walk seamlessly. Avoid outdoor clothing with seams around the shoulders. That's where you'll be intercepting most of the rain if you get caught in a storm. Opt for seams that are tape-sealed. They offer the best protection.

At a Formal Affair

Dressed to Thrill

Proms, then weddings. When it comes to regular guys and tuxedos, that's usually the end of the story. Tuxes are only for Dean Martin and Fred Astaire types, right?

Wrong.

"Any white-collar man over 30 who lives in a major metropolitan area should have a tuxedo in his closet," says Jack Springer, executive director of the International Formalwear Association in Chicago.

"Owning a tux will pay for itself many times over. When you buy one, you're telling yourself that you've arrived in life. When you wear one, you're showing the world that your image is special to you," Springer says.

And when you're not . . . ?

"You're showing the world that you couldn't afford it or, worse, that you didn't care."

Playing the Gussied-Up Game

True, Springer's job is to convince people to buy tuxedos. But there's truth in what he says.

"Imagine going to a formal affair and not dressing appropriately. You'd be mistaken for the help," says image consultant Ken Karpinski.

Most men have never thought about buying a tuxedo of their own. But according to the experts, the black-tie wardrobe—even if it's just one tux—is as important as the corporate wardrobe.

"If you're on the fast track and you think that you're going to climb the ladder, there are going to be occasions where a tuxedo will be absolutely necessary because almost every business has at least one formal function a year," Springer says. "And where I live in Chicago, for example, the social season kicks off with the film festival openings, the opera, and the symphony. They're all black-tie."

The key is the magic phrase "black tie encouraged." That means that it's (hint, hint) a formal affair, but you won't be kicked out for wearing a nice suit. If that's the case, it really means (hint, hint) that black tie is *not* optional.

"The definition of being well-dressed means wearing the right thing in the right place at the right time with the right people," says David Wolfe of The Doneger Group.

Ironically, when the tuxedo was born, it wasn't any of the above. The tux made its debut in 1886 when a socialite showed up at a formal ball held in Tuxedo Park, New York, wearing a short, square, black jacket that resembled a smoking jacket. Because he was well-connected—and because the trendy Prince of Wales was wearing something similar halfway around the world—the socialite wasn't shown the door. Instead, people were soon talking about (and wearing) the "Tuxedo jacket."

As if all this isn't enough to sell you on the value of the tux, consider that:

- 64 percent of women say that a man in a tux looks sexier than a man in a suit
- 55 percent of American men say that they feel more attractive in a tux
- 75 percent of women agree that tuxedos attract more attention than suits

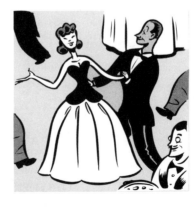

Paint It Black-Tie

In case you haven't figured it out, a formal function is more important style-wise than heading to church, a wedding, or a friend's dinner party. Going to the chairman's ball, a diplomatic dinner, or a formal award banquet is where image counts most.

"Formal affairs are where you're seen to be seen. The key to your image there is how you rack up points," says Princess Jenkins of Majestic Images International. Here's how to make all the right moves when you're back in black.

Dress appropriately. *Always* opt for black-tie apparel when the invitation says "formal" or "black tie optional." For a maximum-style man, it's not a choice.

Understand too that black-tie attire isn't the most formal. White-tie is. When something's white-tie, it's ultra-special. You can imagine the gasps of shock that went up when the fashion public learned that then-President Jimmy Carter's inauguration was a black-tie, not white-tie, event.

Make the call: Buy or rent. If a formal affair is on your agenda, decide whether you want to rent or buy your outfit. If you're renting, most of your problems are solved: You'll be measured, fitted, and outfitted all at once. Of course, you'll also be wearing what every high school senior is wearing to his prom that year. If you buy, pick a traditional, conservative style that will be around forever, and spend as much as you would on a fine suit.

"The thing about a tux is that it doesn't have to be prohibitively expensive. The rule of thumb is that it should cost no more than the suits that you wear," Springer says.

Choose your style. Tuxes come in an array of styles, colors, and cuts. Your basic choice is single- or double-breasted jackets. Single-breasted styles have been around for 100 years and aren't losing ground, says Karpinski. Double-breasted jackets are a little more powerful, but are sometimes dubbed

Why Black Is Beautiful

Two centuries ago, when society's powerhouses wanted to dress up, they chose the brightest colors in the closet. We were a society of peacocks. Fast-forward to today and formalwear is far less flamboyant. The modern colors of choice are black and white.

Why the change? The rage for the charcoal color ironically began with charcoal. Around the early 1800s, well-heeled men in England, then the fashion center of the West, wore black because their industrial cities were so sooty. Only the very rich could afford lighter colors, presumably because only they could keep those clothes clean. Well-to-do, middle-class men pragmatically wore black because it wasn't so high-maintenance. As the middle class expanded and more people discovered its practicality, black naturally stuck.

passé. They also limit your leeway in wearing a cummerbund or vest because they remain buttoned all night. As for color, always pick black. It'll never go out of style.

Tread carefully with color. Formal daywear, especially in warmer climates, allows for lighter-weight and lighter-colored jackets, including white dinner jackets. This is about the only time that white jackets are permissible.

Read the lapel. Tux lapels come in three basic designs: the shawl collar, the peaked collar, and the notched collar. Notched lapels are the most common and conservative. Peaked lapels are often found on double-breasted suits but can look a little overpowering on smaller men. Shawl collars are usually found on dinner jackets and are ultra-traditional and even a little stodgy. Nevertheless, notched and shawl collars will never go out of style.

Be shirt-shape. Tuxedo shirts are white, with or without an accordion-like bib of ruffles. (These pleats come in 5- and 10-pleat varieties.) Although fancier shirts exist, including shirts with patterns, stripes, and colors, you can't go wrong with the tried-and-true, especially on the dressiest occasion.

The tux collar traditionally was a straight collar, though the wing tip has picked up in popularity in recent years. Not every expert feels the same about whether the wing tips go in front of or behind the tie. Springer suggests behind because it shows your tie better.

Banded-collar shirts are another option. Worn without a bow tie, they're not strictly formal.

Choose a cummerbund or vest. Vests are relatively new in formalwear. They're a little more aesthetically pleasing than cummerbunds, though the latter are the traditional favorites. The advantage of a vest is that you can take your jacket off and still look dressy. It also gives you more latitude to express your own style, since vests come in a multitude of colors and patterns.

Be adventurous with accessories. Occasion permitting, you're free to jazz up your duds with accessories. "It's sometimes the only individuality that you can express," says Leon Hall of International Apparel Mart and The Fashion Association, and a frequent fashion commentator and trend forecaster.

Necessary accessories include cuff links and studs for your shirt. Gold with black onyx works well with anything, though you can up the ante with diamond or precious stones, as your budget permits. Other formal accessories you may want to try include bow ties, expensive watches, pocket squares, and braces, which are the buttons on the inside of your pants that hold your trousers up. No one

normally sees your braces, but Karpinski remembers one man, a groom, who decorated his with pink naked angels. He made a divine statement on his wedding night.

Don't be a heel. The right shoes are essential to your outfit. Think nothing less than spit-shined, patent leathers that would make a Marine sergeant proud. Barring that, professionally polished, very plain cap-toe oxfords work in a pinch. As for socks, lightweight fabric, always black, and always mid-calf.

Can the cane and top hat. "These are pretty much regarded as costume props these days," says Springer. "So if you're not in a play or can't tap-dance like Fred Astaire, don't do it."

Preserve your prized wardrobe. Take care of your black-tie wardrobe. Keep a freshly cleaned and pressed tux hanging in your closet in a garment bag or under plastic covering. Put your tux shirt along with it on a hanger, and your patent leathers under it in a soft cloth bag to keep them from getting scratched and becoming dust magnets, Karpinski recommends.

Dressed to the Nines

You say that someone is "dressed to the nines" when he's sporting his very best. This doesn't make much sense at face value, but it's an old saying with an interesting, albeit nebulous, history.

"Dressed to the nines" probably started out as something like "dressed well from head to toe." Since that didn't exactly roll off the tongue, it was probably cut short to "dressed to the eyes," say Graham Donaldson and Sue Setterfield in their book Why Do We Say That? In medieval England, that would have been "dressed to the eyne." Over centuries, misunderstanding and miscommunication and more than a handful of mealymouthed people likely turned "eyne" to "nine."

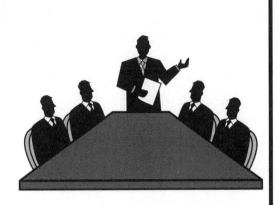

Part Five

Real-Life Scenarios

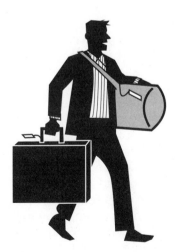

Quest for the Best
These highly successful and celebrated men have reached the pinnacle of their professions. And they've done it without compromising their individual styles. Here are their stories.

You Can Do It!
Just like you, these guys have struggled to maintain their individuality in the face of subtle—and even not-so-subtle—pressure to conform. They've managed to pull it off. So can you.

Stylish to the End
In life, they set the standards for maximum style. And death has done nothing to diminish the lasting impact they had.

Quest for the Best These highly successful and celebrated men have reached the pinnacle of their professions. And they've done it without compromising their individual styles. Here are their stories.

John Peterman, President and Co-Founder, The J. Peterman Company

Style and Simplicity

John Peterman has never appeared on the hit TV comedy show *Seinfeld*. But that hasn't stopped the mail-order clothing company president from becoming a recurring character on the program.

Like New York Yankees owner George Steinbrenner, Peterman found himself caricatured on the show on a regular basis after Elaine—the character played by actress Julia Louis-Dreyfus—went to work for The J. Peterman Company. "It has its pluses and minuses," Peterman muses. "On the plus side, 37 million people are hearing my name; on the minus side, the guy on the show portrays me as a jerk."

But Peterman handles the farcical portrayal with the same self-confidence that allowed him to build a $50 million business from a single cowboy duster. "To tell you the truth, I rarely think about clothes or what people will think of me or my clothes," Peterman says. "I just pick things that I like, and I expect others to do the same. And if you're enough of an individual, it won't matter what clothes you're wearing."

Express Yourself

The seasonal catalogs put out by The J. Peterman Company, called the Owner's Manual, are a testament to Peterman's eclectic individual tastes. The catalogs are filled with detailed watercolors of chamois shirts and fireman's coats, baseball jackets and four-wale corduroy pants. Clothes that every man looks good in because they are "filled with romance," he says.

"Clearly, people want things that make their lives the way they wish they were," Peterman writes in the company's "Philosophy," which is printed on the inside-cover page of each Owner's Manual.

"Amelia Earhart said that before she became a pilot she went out to the airfield and saw that the other guys wore khaki pants and leather jackets," Peterman says. "So she got khakis and leathers and put grease on them. She said that she pretended to become a pilot and then she did become a pilot. It's true for all of us. We pretend and then we become."

But lest you miss the point of the anecdote, remember that Earhart really was, deep down inside, a pilot. If she had tried to

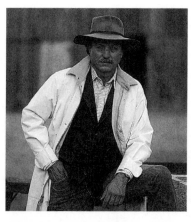

dress the part of a glamour girl, she would have probably never looked stylish. "The same is true for men," says Peterman. "You have to be an individual. You have to be yourself."

That's why you'll find baseball jackets in the catalog. A former professional minor league baseball player, the jackets are a part of Peterman's past. "They evoke a feeling," he says. "When I was a kid, wearing a baseball jacket made a person feel special. Then, you go through a stage in life where you don't wear a baseball jacket, and suddenly you arrive at an age when you would like a little piece of the past. Then the baseball jacket becomes more important to you because it brings you back to that special feeling."

Or perhaps it gives you a special feeling because you've always dreamed about playing baseball. It's dreams that Peterman sells. He started his company in 1987 because so many strangers stopped to ask him where he'd gotten one of his coats, an authentic cowboy duster. He bought 500 of the items, advertised in *The New Yorker* and the *Wall Street Journal*, and quickly sold out. "It was the real thing," Peterman says of the duster that started it all. "That's what's so attractive about it. It's authentic."

Keep It Simple

That commitment to authenticity is the guiding principle behind Peterman's offerings. Genuine Irish sweaters, the David Niven blazer, a Norwegian anorak, the Mission: Impossible trench coat, and, yes, a Pamplona beret are all found within the pages of an Owner's Manual.

Although all these clothes evoke a different mood, class, and history, they share one commonality. "Simplicity," says Peterman. "Style is simplicity, and simple is wonderful and elegant and sophisticated. Anything that varies from simple is not stylish. Simple doesn't mean, however, natural. It's something that you aim for. Nothing in the world comes naturally, although everyone would like to believe that you're just born that way. But we all work at simplicity."

In fact, Peterman adds, people who don't work at simplicity are not his kind of people at

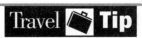

Travel Tip

"As seasoned a traveler as I am, I still take more than I should," says John Peterman of The J. Peterman Company. **"And even though you can buy good stuff wherever you're going, there are still some places where you have to bring everything that you need. Finding underwear in La Paz, Bolivia, is difficult, for example."**

What's Peterman's best advice for the international traveler? **"Try not to look like an American or a tourist,"** he says. **"Wear the same kind of clothes that everyone else is wearing."** Hey! Doesn't this contradict his theory that we should all strive to be individuals? **"Well, there can be a penalty for being an individual in some places,"** says Peterman. **"You should be respectful in another country because you're the foreigner."**

That's just the reality of traveling, he says, and even an old romantic like him struggles with reality.

"If I had my druthers, I'd like to send a steamer trunk ahead and have it in my room when I arrived at the hotel," he fantasizes. **"I'd come in and all my suits would be hung up in a closet. My black tux would be there, ready to go. One of these days I'm going to do that."**

For now, though, Peterman has his own style of packing. **"I take a soft-side duffel bag wherever I go,"** he says. **"I even pack my suits and sport jacket in it. I just lay the pants on the bottom, and that keeps them pressed."**

all. "I have an instant distrust for anyone who is too flashy," Peterman says. "If you're insecure, you want flashy, loud clothes; but if you're secure, you want to make another kind of statement. Everything we choose, from clothes to cars, we choose to make a statement. The art is being able to pull it off."

And how does Peterman want to feel? Romantic.

Ed Bradley, *60 Minutes* Reporter

"What You See Is What You Get"

Ed Bradley comes on the small screen every Sunday on CBS and we immediately see a fellow spirit. The veteran *60 Minutes* reporter is on our side, the good guys' side. We are magnetized by the image of this big burly person with the bushy salt-and-pepper beard, the tiny earring, the bold wardrobe, and the knowing eyes with a twinkle of mischief in the corners.

There is something almost contradictory about him: on one hand a sympathetic smile that makes you want to sip cognac by a fire and reveal all your vulnerabilities, on the other a take-no-prisoners journalist who would spend all night unearthing some document to betray you.

"Ed is the embodiment of integrity," says Diane Sawyer, anchor of *PrimeTime Live*, the hour-long weekly magazine on ABC, and long-time friend and colleague of Bradley. Reminding us that the word *integrity* means "wholeness," she goes on: "His style, his eternally hip walk, and his power are direct expressions of the authentic man inside. Nothing phony. Nothing for show. Everything his alone."

That is probably why *TV Guide* readers voted him second-most competent, fourth-most intelligent, and fourth-most trusted man in TV news. (For the record, Walter Cronkite ranked first in every category but most attractive.)

Bradley offers his own explanation for this vote of confidence: "People feel that I'm fair. I'm not vindictive in my interviewing style and technique. I try to get at the information. If I'm beating up on someone, it's because they deserve to be beat up on. And I think that I have a track record that vindicates their trust in me."

He certainly does: 11 Emmys, 4 Alfred Dupont/

Columbia University citations, 1 George Foster Peabody award, 1 George Polk award, and 3 Overseas Press Club awards.

Despite all this, however, there is a modesty, a one-of-us quality that he reveals in this anecdote: "Over my computer I keep a picture of me standing at the Khyber Pass in Afghanistan. I can remember when that was taken, thinking about the history of the area, of Alexander the Great going through here, thinking"—and here, he breaks into a voice reminiscent of Bradley's friend and CBS colleague Bill Cosby recounting one of his treasured boyhood memories—"Wow, 'Butch' Bradley (that was my nickname) from West Philly at the Khyber Pass. The same thing happened on the Great Wall of China. I hope I never lose that appreciation of those wow moments. If I do, then it's time to do something else."

Keeping His Cool

His auspicious career started in an inauspicious manner—as a jazz disc jockey on radio station WDAS in Philadelphia. "That was my initial attraction," he says. "I did the news to get my foot in the door." He ended up as FM program director there—in charge of one other staffer and himself. (For pure pleasure, he still hosts a radio show, *Jazz at Lincoln Center*, on National Public Radio.)

Generally speaking, he says, his on-camera persona is not that different from the person that you would meet off camera: "In many ways, what you see is what you get."

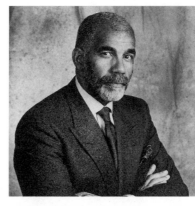

On camera, even in the midst of the classic *60 Minutes* "I gotcha" moments—when the evidence stacked in front of the public official forces him to admit incompetence or even wrongdoing—Bradley maintains his cool, the perfect poker player. "I never show my anger on camera," he explains. "It gets in the way of the purpose of being there in the first place: to get some information or clarify a situation. If you lose control, you've lost. You have to stay focused on what it is you're after and keep moving ahead."

He applies that same tactic to his personal style. But remembering is not always easy in the heat of the moment, he admits: "My anger is more inner than outer. I get quiet when I get angry. When anger is justified, it's better to say, 'I'm angry and upset, and I'd like to talk about it.' My tendency often is to sit on things—and I have to work on it."

One of the ways he blows off steam from journalism's intense, deadline-ridden world is with a rigorous exercise regime and getaways to his ski cabin in Colorado. A hair under six feet one inch and in a continual struggle to keep his weight "under rather than over 200 pounds," he tries "doing something aerobic every day," including workouts on his stair-climber at home and a stretching program.

Bradley takes equal care in how he drapes that body. He prides himself in dressing well and clearly enjoys talking men's fashion. He buys "off the rack" from Armani and other big-name designers. The world is literally his shopping mall. There's a place in San Francisco that he goes back to all the time. He frequents a clothier in London. At another shop, whenever he's in Hong Kong, he has shirts tailor-made.

His personal dressing style runs to bold patterns in ties, anything in rich shades of the colors blue, gray, and earthy brown and fine looking fabrics. Understated but creative.

The pierced ear is barely noticeable on camera and hardly mentionable if he weren't a reporter for a major television network. "It's true," he says. "I'm probably the only network news guy with an earring." To Bradley, however, it's no big statement. "Some people notice it. Some don't. Some like it. Some don't. I

Travel Tip

CBS newsman Ed Bradley estimates that he logs about 500,000 miles a year. Here are some inside scoops from a seasoned traveler.

Make a list. "If I don't list what I plan to wear every day, and then pack accordingly, right down to socks, inevitably I'll screw it up," he says. Despite his best intentions, sometimes he overpacks. "I'd rather have too much than too little," he explains.

Express yourself. He tries to pack only enough to bring carry-on baggage. If he sees that he's going over, he'll spend the extra money to send them ahead by Express Mail. "Then it's at the hotel when I get there," he says. He recommends the same for us common Joes if the time lost waiting for baggage to come off the carousel is more profitably spent rushing to your first appointment right from the airport.

Take a mini-vacation. "Always take a book and some of your favorite music," he suggests. He finds that disappearing into a good book or a choice tape or CD creates some distance from the hubbub, "and it keeps you in touch with yourself," he adds.

---

wanted to do it for a few years. I thought that it would be cool. That's all."

Being with *60 Minutes* since 1980, Bradley looks neither back nor forward but seems to enjoy the present moment. "I have no idea what I'll do next," he says. "I'm not the kind of person who makes long-range plans. The first time CBS wanted me to sign to a five-year contract, I balked."

But true to Bradley style, we'll get to continue identifying with the sympathetic do-gooder on *60 Minutes* "as long as it's fun," he says. "When it stops being fun, I'll look for something else that's fun."

Robert Palmer, Musician

Addicted to Style

The son of a British naval officer, rock singer Robert Palmer learned at an early age the importance of dressing stylishly.

"I grew up in Malta, a group of islands south of Sicily, and it was an international, mostly naval society. My parents used to take me out to swell evenings," Palmer recalls. "It was up to the guests to guess who was the best-dressed. Even then I recognized that some people had flair."

In a pop culture dominated by the uniform of flannel, T-shirts, and jeans, Palmer stands out as a man of impeccable style and taste. Since he launched into the pop music scene in the 1970s—and particularly since his groundbreaking music video of the early 1980s, "Addicted to Love"—Palmer has projected an image of cool sophistication. It fits him like one of his expensive Italian suits. "I don't think my look is a contrivance," he says. "I just can't think of a more comfortable alternative."

Palmer, however, doesn't dress to impress others. "Actually, I just really enjoy the quality of a good tailor's work, or a good cobbler's work," he says. "Sometimes I just see a pair of shoes and go, 'Whoa!'"

For Palmer, good style is defined by appropriateness. "I think about the week ahead and try to plan my wardrobe," he says. "Usually, I have a rehearsal and some interviews, and I always have to ask myself, 'What can I carry with me?' since my efforts these days carry me around the world."

Palmer usually travels with a couple of suits, a casual outfit, and "something to get there and back in." Which, it should come as no surprise, is usually a suit. In fact, to Palmer "casual" means a jacket and slacks, especially trousers that don't crease.

"I'm comfortable in a jacket and tie," says Palmer. "If it's Texas and 100°F, I don't wear a tie, but if it's Prague and it's freezing, then I do. While the essence of style is to be appropriate for the situation, I don't dress down." As a rule, he doesn't wear jeans unless he's hiking in the woods. "I think that women can more likely carry off a pair of jeans because of their poise and makeup," Palmer says. "Men tend to look scruff.

"I lived in the Bahamas for a few years, and it was considered a luxury to have air-conditioning. But I had it installed so that I could have parties and get dressed up," Palmer says. "I look forward to winter so that I can wear my favorite clothes."

Mr. Mannequin

Yes, Palmer says, he has a lot of clothes. "Although I see a lot of things that I don't buy because I don't need them," he adds. Palmer shops in Milan, which is only an hour away from his home in Switzerland. Because he has been shopping in the same designer stores for 15 years, salespeople tend to hold on to suits that they know Palmer will like. "In Milan the designers make up a set of things for the runway, and I'm just lucky that

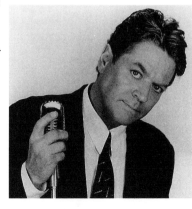

they happen to be my size," says Palmer. "And it isn't as if they hold bizarre items. It's usually just a casual suit."

Because Palmer buys from the designer, the suits cost less. "Instead of the suit costing $4,000 in needless markup, I usually pay $500. And it's a one-of-a-kind item," he explains.

Can't get to Milan? Palmer advises other lovers of

fine clothes to find out which designer's suits fit them the best. "I'm Mr. Mannequin. The prototypes of certain designers, such as Ferre and Armani, just happen to fit me," he explains. "And, the most important thing about shopping is to have something in mind before you go looking."

Palmer's main indulgence is shirts. "A man can't have enough white shirts," he says. "Although they are basically all the same. I buy them two sizes too big, and in three months they're too tight from the laundry and I throw them away."

Does he look back at his numerous videos and TV performances and see any fashion faux pas? "No, I only run the risk of being boring," says Palmer. "The suit I wore in the 'Addicted to Love' video is my own, and, in fact, I have two of them that I still wear. It's just a nice gray suit that makes me feel as if I'm dressed invisibly."

Terrance Donovan, the director of the video, was familiar with Palmer's clothing style when he conceived of the video's look. "Basically, he said, 'Trust me, be there at 4:00 P.M.,' and I flew in from somewhere looking like I usually do," Palmer recounts. "I mimed the tune in front of a blue screen and flew back home to the Bahamas.

"I don't want to be noticed. Instead, I dress conservatively and formally," he says. "But since I'm hardly like that in person, I do run the risk of being a wolf in sheep's clothing." Of the many rock stars who dress for attention, Palmer thinks that David Lee Roth pulls it off the best. "David Lee Roth is sort of the epitome of rock and roll bravado. Most people would look ridiculous dressed the way he does, but he carries it off very well. I think that he's very stylish and he's quite comfortable with the stares from other people."

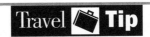

Travel Tip

"If you're traveling for business, buy the best," rock singer Robert Palmer advises. "There really is a difference in how well a suit can travel." If you're wearing sneakers, jeans, and a T-shirt, the quality doesn't matter, but if you have to stand in front of people soon after your flight, then you want to look your best, he adds.

Half the time, Palmer says, musicians get off a plane, leave the airport, go into a theater through the back door, and get right up on stage without even knowing what city they're in. "You can't see them, but they can see you," he says of the audience. "I never understood the point of dressing down. I didn't understand it when I opened for The Who when I was 16, and I don't understand it now."

The Finishing Touches

Palmer wears cologne because he enjoys fragrance, not because he thinks that it's a necessity. He prefers Givenchy and Van Cleef and Arpels. "However, good grooming really does indicate if someone cares about himself. It's a matter of basic self-respect," says Palmer. "I really appreciate people who look after themselves, male or female, but it has to be normal and natural, not artificial or overdone."

While some people carry off the American clothing styles of cowboy boots and baseball caps excellently, says Palmer, he dislikes the uniformity of those types of clothes. Because he's confident in his own sense of style, Palmer remains unconcerned about what everyone else is wearing. So what would he do if he woke up tomorrow morning and found that everyone was wearing a gray suit?

"I'd applaud," he says.

Isadore Sharp, Founder, Chairman, and CEO, Four Seasons/Regent Hotels and Resorts

Hotelier with Haute Style

Style of the five-star variety is all attitude in the hotel world, says Isadore Sharp. The man should know. As founder, chairman, and chief executive officer of what is arguably the world's best upscale hotel management chain, he has instilled in his employees—in some 40 hotels in 16 countries throughout the world—an attitude that has raised the stakes of style in the hospitality industry.

Sure, you have to have the top-tier hardware and the software in place. But then it's all about "a moment of contact," says the wiry six-footer, who everyone knows as Issy. "It starts with motivating our staff to making a commitment to caring. I encourage the idea that 99 percent customer satisfaction is not enough. So even though perfection is an ever-receding goal, we are in pursuit of it all the time."

That's it. No secret formula. No fancy marketing. Just the human touch. "More than any other hotelier that I have worked with or for, Issy has a way of bringing out the best in people," says veteran hotelier Stan Bromley, previously with Hyatt Hotels and now a Four Seasons regional vice-president and general manager of the company's prestigious Washington, D.C., property.

While other luxury hotel chains in the United States have adapted the upscale stodgy style in the tradition of the formal grand hotels of Europe, Sharp believed that North Americans

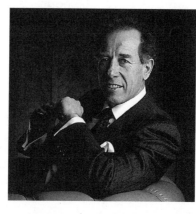

wanted something a bit more casual without compromising on quality. He hires people based not on how well they can serve a drink or make a bed but on their friendliness and their cooperativeness.

The Sharp approach to style has paid off. Through 1996, the hotels that come under the banner of the Four Seasons/Regent Canadian flag have won more coveted Five Diamond Awards from the American Automobile Association than any other hotel company. In 1996 reader surveys by *Conde Nast Traveler*, *Institutional Investor*, and *Travel and Leisure*, the company reaped more honors than any other hotel group.

Company revenues hover under $200 million a year. With his investment in the company, Sharp's worth has been estimated to be more than $100 million.

Rags to Riches

Sharp's success is rather remarkable for the son of a poor Polish couple that immigrated to Canada from what was then the Jewish state of Palestine. Known as Razzle-Dazzle Issy on the basketball court in college, young Sharp also played collegiate football and ice hockey at Ryerson Polytechnic University in Toronto. After earning a degree in architecture in 1952, he worked his way up through his father's small construction company. He caught the hotel bug after building a small motor inn for a Canadian couple. Big on visions of what he would do if he could build his own hotel— but short on cash when no bank would back the unproven entrepreneur—he convinced his brother-in-law (a successful furrier) and the founder of a major drugstore chain to put up $180,000 to his own $90,000. This first foray into hotels, at age 30, was North America's first "motor hotel" in 1961, built in a less-than-desirable section of Toronto. The best room at that first Four Seasons Hotel, a replica of a medieval castle with interior courtyard and swimming pool, went for $12.50 per night.

From that first hotel, a "Four Seasons" style evolved. "We never wanted to create a cookie-cutter experience," he says now. "Each hotel has its own look, its own style."

Sharp, now in his mid-sixties, credits the development of his own sense of style to his wife, Rosalie, an interior designer who has been involved in the look of a number of Four Seasons properties. "She had me wearing colorful print ties 15 years before they were in," he recalls. "I've picked up her style by osmosis."

While they both laugh about how many expensive Italian suits and fine thin-soled Italian leather shoes now cram his closet, she points to something else about him that has more to do with his own interior design. "His style comes from within him," she says. "Issy is a sweetheart. He has a sweet soul, and that's the reason why people swoon over him when he comes into a room." Not to mention that "he has the body of an 18-year-old," she swoons herself.

He keeps his athletic body in shape by exercising four or five times a week to one of Jane Fonda's original advanced aerobic tapes, but that soulful compassionate side of him comes naturally. A strong financial supporter of Jewish causes and many other community charities, he is most proud of his leadership role in the Terry Fox Run, which honors the efforts of a young Canadian who lost first a leg and then his life to cancer. When Fox staged a cross-country run to raise awareness and money to fight the spread of cancer, the Sharps, who had lost a son to the disease, were there with financial support from the start. The annual event, of which Sharp is director, now takes place

in 55 countries and is approaching the $200 million mark of total funds raised toward the cause.

Sharp expects the same from those who work for him. "I believe as a company that we are responsible to the community," he says. "So I make sure that everybody in the company does *something* of a charitable or philanthropic nature."

Travel Tip

One would suspect that a man who sells sleep would have some good advice up his well-tailored sleeve on how to get a night's rest for those who check into hotels only occasionally. One would suspect correctly. Here are the best tips for all seasons from Isadore Sharp of Four Seasons/Regent Hotels.

Start with a quiet room. "Any noise that is unusual from your normal experience is going to seem too loud in a foreign environment," Sharp says. Ask for a room facing the quiet side of the hotel. If the fan on the air conditioning or heating system is too loud, turn it off.

Bounce on the bed. Before you decide to take the room, make sure that the bed is as firm or as soft as you like. "There is nothing more intimate than one's bed, and it's key to a sound sleep," says Sharp.

Take control of your environment. If you like to breathe fresh air when you sleep, make sure that you know how to open the windows (if they open at all). Know where the thermostat is and how to use it. Find the extra blanket (usually hidden on the closet shelf) *before* you bed down for the night. If you don't find it, have one sent up.

Stay in the dark. Make sure that your shades are drawn tightly, checking to see that one side overlaps the other and the ends reach the walls. Those little rays of light will seem like floodlights in the morning.

Ric Flair, Professional Wrestler

It's His Nature to Be Stylish

Ric Flair is an unexpected epicure in the philistine world of professional wrestling. At six feet one inch, 240 pounds, the platinum-blond Flair stands out in any crowd. But among colleagues who make their mark by cracking skulls and shouting threats, Flair's polish and panache are even more distinguishing.

When he's not smashing opponents with a Flying Knee Drop or ensnaring them in his infamous Figure Four leglock, Flair generally can be found ringside, wearing a tuxedo, sipping champagne, and being mobbed by beautiful women. He plays the role of Nature Boy—his most popular nickname—with a natural flair. "I've always liked clothes and admired people who dress well," Flair says. "My playboy image was easy for me. It's what people want, so it's easy to play off of.

"People want fame and fortune. They want the finer things in life, and they respect someone who has that," Flair says. "That's all the stuff that I brag about. It was only four years ago that I stopped wearing a suit every day."

Flair established his wrestling image early on. It was a fun lifestyle, one that meshed with his own wild side and, most important, one that appealed to his fans. As with most fashion mavens, Flair perches on the leading edge most of the time. Looking back, he says, he occasionally wound up on the bleeding edge.

"I used to wear a lot of jewelry when jewelry was hot for guys, and real flashy clothes," he laughs.

His wife, Beth, reminds him about the colored lizard shoes. And the gaudy jewelry. And the Mr. T–style gold chains. And orange and blue plaid suits.

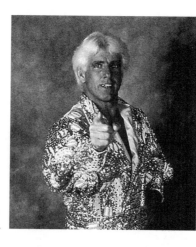

"I figured that he was a pimp, because I wasn't sure why else all these women were around him when he was dressed like that," she says.

"Yeah, I guess you could say that I've toned it down a bit now," Flair adds. "My wife is still correcting me and telling me what not to wear sometimes. She actually buys a lot of my stuff."

He did, however, manage to escape one fashion disaster basically unscathed. He admits to wearing bell bottoms "maybe once or twice, but I never really went that route."

A Familiar Ring

Born Richard Morgan Fliehr in Minneapolis, Flair is the son of a physician father and theater activist mother. Flair never thought about becoming a professional wrestler, even though he watched wrestling on TV and enjoyed it as a kid. He became a wrestler around his sophomore year in college. "Let's say that I never predicted my grade point average that year," he says.

Flair left school at the University of Minnesota and began selling insurance. Thanks to great athletic conditioning in his youth and to wrestling and playing football for the university, he vaulted into professional wrestling after meeting and teaming up with Verne Gagne and later Greg "The Hammer" Valentine. "Selling life insurance was something that I did to feed myself until wrestling camp started," he says. "It was through necessity, not design, and it was either that or tend bar. Since I was already a bar bouncer and still needed extra money, insurance helped pay the bills."

Flair started out strong in his new career, apparently having been born with a flair for professional grappling. He and his tag-team partners won their early matches, and the rest is history. Flair has since been a world champion 13 times over, and has won every title in the sport.

Today, Flair resides in Charlotte, North Carolina. He has lived there since 1975, with his wife and four children, two from a previous marriage. Much of his time, when he's not wrestling, is spent running a string of seven successful Gold's Gyms, which he owns and operates. Like many of us, he struggles with familial duties and work-related travel.

"I dread the traveling. I used to love it, but now all that it is is time away from the family," he says. "I'm as obsessed now about being the best father and businessman I can as I was with being the best wrestler."

Although Flair has settled down considerably, he's still a stickler for image and style. "I like to call it image enhancement," he says. "Image is everything, especially when you're on TV. Being able to sell yourself is what separates the men from the boys.

"One thing that's been an asset to me is the fact that I've always been Ric Flair. A lot of guys, especially in this sport, go through identity crises and change their images," Flair says. "I never have. I am Ric Flair, I've always been Ric Flair, and I'll always be Ric Flair. I think that people appreciate that."

Fans will appreciate Flair's future plans, too. They're as steady as his identity: He intends to continue wrestling until he's no longer a leading contender. "I want to remain in the top five," he says. "Not the five most popular wrestlers but the top five best wrestlers. As long as I feel that I'm in the top five best wrestlers, I'll stay full steam ahead."

Flair also plans to stay on course with healthy living and exercise. Fitness for Flair is his most enduring form of image enhancement. "Of all the gimmicks that have come and gone over the years, fitness and good health are the

Travel 🧳 Tip

Professional wrestler Ric Flair spends more than 300 days a year on the road. He has racked up more than 2.2 million frequent-flier miles on Delta Airlines alone. Here's what he has learned.

Get an agent. "The greatest travel tip that I can pass on is to have a really informed, educated, professional travel agent. Someone who can be there for you in two seconds and have the cars, trains, planes, and hotels ready," Flair says. "Travel is so much easier when you're organized, and your trip home has to be as enjoyable and efficient as your departure."

Pass time productively. "The hardest part of traveling is battling the lines. It doesn't happen as much to celebrities, to be honest, but it happens. I read. *Sports Illustrated, Men's Health, People Weekly.* Magazines. Lots of magazines. I bring four or five."

Enjoy the ride. "Airline flight crews really want you to enjoy your flight. If I'm not reading, I try to make the most of what they offer. I'll listen to the in-flight music once in a while, but what I enjoy most, besides reading, is trying to get into the in-flight movie if it's a good one."

longest lasting," he says. "I don't think that will change. The day that someone stops worrying about what he looks like is the day that he has a real problem.

"I understand lack of confidence and how easy it is to procrastinate. Believe me, you can find an excuse for not doing anything in life," Flair says. "But staying in shape and being healthy is important. It's a mental thing as much as it is a physical thing. It's discipline, for the body and mind."

And *that's* maximum style.

You Can Do It! Just like you, these guys have struggled to maintain their individuality in the face of subtle—and even not-so-subtle—pressure to conform. They've managed to pull it off. So can you.

From Sophomore to Savvy

Jonathan Cope, Chicago, Illinois

Date of birth: January 7, 1968

Height and weight: 5-foot-10, 150 pounds

Profession: Corporate lawyer

Throughout most of college, I wore the no-brainer wardrobe. Khakis with button-down blue shirts, khakis with button-down white, and, for a change of pace, khakis with work shirts.

When I graduated and took my first job working for a commercial real estate developer, I looked in my closet and realized that the row of khakis would work for Casual Friday—but nothing else. I went to Fields Department Store in Chicago and splurged on my first suit. I still remember it fondly: It was a dark blue suit, Perry Ellis Portfolio, single-button. I paid $350, put it on a credit card, and paid it off the next month.

Law school was an education in what not to wear if you become an attorney. People don't care what they wear—they hardly shower. Even the professors were not overly concerned with their attire. Part of what nobody tells you but that you figure out is that each firm has its own dress code. You were, therefore, on your own in choosing clothing for clerkship interviews. Many of the larger firms fall into the conservative category. They'd sooner have their academic records stand out than their ties. Show up for an interview in a flashy outfit, and you've blown your chances. So it was with great care that I picked out and bought the suit

that I wore for my first law firm interview. It was a Joseph Abboud. I paid about $400.

Now I work for a 300-attorney corporate law firm in downtown Chicago. It has a reputation as a younger firm with aggressive entrepreneurial personalities. Men dress pretty fashionably: pinstripe Italian-cut suits, striped and colored shirts, pants with cuffs, and high-end loafers.

I came in owning about four suits. Now I have about 10 and I pay as much as $900 a suit. I own probably several thousand dollars' worth of suits, shirts, ties, and shoes. On a lawyer's salary, that's not a small amount—but it's a necessary expenditure. In my profession it's important to look successful.

I generally buy my suits at a men's specialty shop—Syd Jerome's downtown here. Like many busy professionals, I just don't have time to mess around looking through racks of clothes.

I defer to his judgment. I put my faith in him. When he starts to get a little too flashy, I have to rein him back in. Now I'll wear a spread-collar white shirt, Pat Riley–style, with a flowered-type patterned Donna Karan tie, and a dark blue Zegna suit.

I've learned some of the ingredients that help you put your own look together. He's taught me a lot. I used to think that a shirt was a shirt. You either wore white or blue. And I have several colors of suits—solid gray and gray pinstripe, blue, taupe, and a couple of others in both double- and single-breasted. Now I'm a little more savvy. And I've come to really enjoy looking well-dressed. Once you get used to dressing in style, it's hard to go back to khakis and blazers.

Banking on Style

Paul F. McAtee, Jr., Glendale, California

Date of birth: September 14, 1942

Height and weight: 6 feet, 180 pounds

Profession: Business consultant/entrepreneur

It's ironic, my background, that is, considering my career and where I am today. I grew up in the Ozarks, deep in Missouri. My father was a railroad worker, and we lived in the woods. I didn't see TV until I was 16, and we didn't have running water or electric lights. From as early as I can remember, I wanted to move to the big city because that's where things were happening. (That's funny, because everybody I know now wants to escape from the city.)

After undergraduate school at the University of Missouri in Columbia and an M.B.A. from Washington University in St. Louis, I moved to California and went into banking. Banking, especially in the early 1970s, was very restrictive. It was the epitome of conservatism. If you hoped to make it, you had to wear the uniform—and I did. My work wardrobe was nothing but dark suits and white shirts. I didn't wear a striped shirt to work until the mid-1980s.

The image of a banker suited me fine for my entire career. I never liked having my style dictated to me, but I'm very conservative by nature, especially as far as dress is concerned, so it worked for me.

I thought that I knew a lot about business when I left banking in the early 1990s and started my own company, the Small Business Growth Association. I did and do, but I still had a lot to learn. In my job now, I advise small businesses worth up to $25 million with anywhere from 1 to 300 employees. That means that I'm dealing with all sorts of people with all sorts of backgrounds, education, and personalities.

At first I did what I was comfortable with. I wore conservative suits and spoke in high-finance terms of margins, return on equity, and forecasting. My friends who were my first clients told me that they had no idea what I was talking about. The only thing that they wanted to know was how to make money. Then I became aware of my clothing and the parts of me that were projecting a remote image. I had my colors done, even though I never bought into that stuff, and had my wardrobe reviewed by image consultant Louise Elerding, president of the Association of Image Consultants International and owner of The Color Studio in Glendale, California, with whom I was friendly. It turns out that I was relying on what I liked most, not necessarily what worked best. Just like with me speaking in financial jargon, I was relying on what I was comfortable with and not thinking about whether my clients were comfortable, too. As a result, I was sending messages that I never intended to send.

In the end, I changed my vocabulary, my wardrobe, and my overall approach. To be perfectly honest, I'm delighted with the result. If I'm going to speak to a diversified group of businesspeople, I'll wear a sport coat, slacks, and tie. If I'm talking to a group of lawyers, as I did a month ago, I'll wear a suit. My thought process is different, too. Now I know when to talk in terms of margins and return on equity and when not to. Personally and philosophically, this suits me best because I don't care for pretentious people who use big words to impress others.

I wish that I would have learned all this in grad school. I learned book smarts and how to deal with numbers in school, but I learned people smarts and how to deal with people after school. I've kept my accent, and I'm happy being a plain-speaking Missouri boy. Some people might interpret it as being a redneck, but I play up on the Southern hospitality angle and it can work. I wheel and deal with some of the richest, most powerful businessmen in California and can still go into a bar in the Missouri backwoods and fit in perfectly.

Standing Out in a Crowd

Larry Belt, Philadelphia, Pennsylvania

Date of birth: September 16, 1946

Height and weight: 6-foot-1, 150 pounds

Profession: Clothing buyer

After 20-plus years in the fashion and retail clothing industry, I've grown used to all sorts of dress codes and environments. So when I started my job at The Doneger Group in New York City, I thought that I knew what to expect.

I was wrong.

Somewhere around my third or fourth day of work, I showed up wearing a black turtleneck. I remember coming to work wondering if it was too casual. Granted, I wore it to stick out a wee bit. After all, I was new and I wanted to make the right impression, but I've always been like that: I don't mind drawing attention to myself or creating a tiny bit of controversy. I certainly didn't intend to buck the trend or send the wrong signals, but suffice it to say that early on I was told that turtlenecks wouldn't cut it. Since the dress code isn't likely to change anytime soon to accommodate me, I'm changing, of course, to fit in. I did get attention, that's for sure.

The funny thing about the fashion and clothing industry is that they're much more conservative than people think. Almost everywhere I've worked has been more conservative than my own personal style—not that I'm way out there or on the edge of fashion, but I am distinctive. I've always tried to preserve my individuality while conforming just enough to fit in. That's important to me because there are certain things in life that I won't compromise on. I simply won't let myself step backward on some things, but clothing isn't always one of them. There are ways, as I've discovered, to dress the part while keeping your own taste intact. Today at work, for example, I'll wear shirts and ties. They might be a little more daring, but I'll fit in and still be myself.

And I'll leave the turtleneck at home.

I got into the clothing industry through the back door, actually. I spent two years in the Army—I was drafted, and very lucky that I didn't go to Vietnam—and started in retail as a part-time job at night when I got out. My full-time job was doing sales for a company that sold custom-engineered mining equipment. Huge machines that separated minerals and pulverized things. I don't know why I did it. It certainly didn't appeal to me, so eventually I moved into retail full-time.

For the longest time, I worked on the personnel end. I have a way of managing people. As part of the training process, I moved into operations and found that I loved it. I became a buyer, which means that I buy the products that the store sells, and it was everything I was looking for. You need good people skills in buying. You need to know what the customer wants and what the customer is looking for. The other part of the job is looking ahead to see what's happening trend-wise and to predict what's going to happen next season. The biggest thing, again, is understanding who, what, and where your customer is and what your customer wants and will want.

I guess the most important part of style for me is being myself. Even when I buy merchandise, I find myself not wearing what I'm buying. Certainly not because it's not good enough, but because I don't want to look like what's already there. In the Army there was never any room for expression. Now I like being an individual.

One thing that I think helps me stand out from the crowd, besides clothing, is my sense of humor. Oftentimes what you say on the job isn't particularly interesting, but if you can say it in a way that is, you're ahead of the game. I try to inject humor whenever appropriate. It's good for breaking the ice, and it's good for making whatever I'm saying memorable. Not that I'm rib-tickling all day long, but appropriate humor gets you noticed.

Expressing Yourself in the Corporate Jungle

Neil Tepper, Atlanta, Georgia

Date of birth: October 18, 1942

Height and weight: 5-foot-9½, 138 pounds

Profession: Communications creative director-producer

I was always sort of offbeat. I was named most original in my graduating high school class. The quote under my yearbook picture said, "The apparel oft proclaims the man." I got my flair for clothes from my father, an insurance salesman, who was a real clotheshorse. He dressed impeccably but in a rather traditional style. Of course, I had to go in a different direction, but my dad gave me the basics.

One of my fondest memories was going into Manhattan Saturday mornings to buy clothes from manufacturers in the garment district. We never bought off the rack. I quickly learned that style had nothing to do with money. I developed an eye for original looks that appealed to me as different. I never tried to ride any fashion trend.

Style is about being human, even in the corporate setting. No matter what they're wearing or the title that they hold, people are looking for those moments to show their humanity, to connect. Whatever I wear, whatever title I hold, I try to let that essence come through me.

I believe that I have an ability to empathize with people. I gauge where they're at, find my own comfort level, and then meet them somewhere in between. You have to subtly introduce yourself. If you come in acting like an alien, you'll be resisted. You can't start lighting incense and sitting on your desk in the lotus position. People resist that. Like they resist certain words, like "God" and "love."

It took a while to learn this. My first corporate job was working in marketing for Seagram's on Park Avenue in New York City.

But New York and the corporate setting felt too confining. I hadn't figured out how to define myself in that environment without compromising my identity.

So I quit and moved out west, where the do-your-own-thing philosophy was accepted—even encouraged. Eventually, I ended up in Hawaii doing freelance photography and media consulting. My favorite outfit was a pair of faded green corduroy shorts, a sleeveless T-shirt, and sandals (when I wore anything on my feet). After a couple of years I was ready for the career challenge that could only be found back on the mainland, and I rejoined the corporate world with Coca-Cola in Atlanta.

I have a knack in taking the expected so-called uniform and bending the rules just a bit. When I became creative director in the communications department of Coca-Cola, sneakers were frowned upon. But sometimes in summer I wore this seersucker suit with light blue stripes, a grape-colored tie, a white shirt with subtle purple stripes, and a silk pocket square, with bluish athletic socks and brand new white sneakers. It was a package.

I did the same thing when I went to work as vice-president of creative services for MCA Television, part of the big entertainment conglomerate in Universal City, California. This was Hollywood and everything was supposed to be casual, but I was working for a company whose dress code was like a law office's—strictly conservative suits. Well, I started introducing sweaters into my attire. I'd wear it under my suit and then take the jacket off in the office. I'd wear a denim shirt with a silk tie. Another day I'd wear more casual footwear. But the trick was to return the next day to the fine Italian shoes or whatever. I'd intentionally do something a little different every two or three days and then come back to the dress code so that they'd know that I hadn't gone off the deep end.

My attitude was not to snub authority. It was, "Let's get real." There's always a way to gently widen the parameters, to allow your own personality to shine through.

Stylish to the End In life, they set the standards for maximum style. And death has done nothing to diminish the lasting impact they had.

Cary Grant

His Style Was No Charade

He was born Archibald Alexander Leach, in Bristol, England, in 1904, to a working-class couple. Those humble origins never left him, even long after he had become one of the world's most famous and stylish actors of the twentieth century: Cary Grant.

That ability to transcend his own rough-hewn beginnings are part of what made him so stylish, suggests Barbara Shulgasser, chief film critic for the *San Francisco Examiner* and co-author with director Robert Altman of the screenplay for the 1994 film *Ready to Wear*.

"He's a great example of the difference between being fashionable and having style," says Shulgasser, who interviewed Grant in 1984 ("he was 80 but looked 58," she recalls). "Style is innate. Despite his upbringing, he had the capacity to see and instinctively understand what style is in order to transform himself."

In a film career that spanned more than 30 years—from *This Is the Night* in 1932 to *Walk, Don't Run* in 1966—Cary Grant combined debonair charm, intelligence, and a touch of mischievous humor without ever seeming to get ruffled. In *Charade*, a 1963 film co-starring Audrey Hepburn, he takes a shower, fully clothed, hardly even mussing his hair.

"Being British always adds a touch of class in the American filmgoer's mind, but it's the mix of his gritty background that makes him all the more appealing," agrees Robert Sklar, professor in the Department of Cinema Studies

at New York University's Tisch School of the Arts in New York City and author of several books on film, including *City Boys: Cagney, Bogart, Garfield*. "Plus there was that distinctive accent, neither typical English nor typical American. That unique, almost regal voice became his signature."

Of course, there were other assets: "disturbingly good looks, a dazzling smile, and a disarmingly self-deprecating good humor," adds Shulgasser. Not to mention a chin cleft almost as deep as the Grand Canyon.

She suggests that one of his earliest professional performing experiences, with an acrobatic comedy troupe, helped enhance a "natural grace that was physical as well as deeply aesthetic.

"He said that he learned what it meant to be cool under pressure from the great George Burns," she continues. "He learned how to have surface calmness, how to move through the air with total self-control."

On-screen, he had this gesture—a little shrug and raised eyebrows—"that to me reflects his appreciation about how unimportant each of us is that I think made him so attractive, as though he understands that he's a little fish in a huge pond," Shulgasser says.

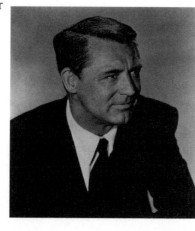

But it was his gentlemanly charm offscreen that drew women to him like moths to a flame. Even film critics. "After my profile of him came out, he called to thank me and tell me that it was one of the best on him that he had read," she recalls. "This was someone who had had thousands of articles written about him. He didn't have to do that. But that's what 'Cary Grant' did."

John F. Kennedy

Setting the Style for a Nation

It was Valentine's Day 1962. The financially beleaguered Studebaker car company posted an unexpected 20-cent-a-share profit. Goodyear Tire and Rubber Company profits climbed to record levels. Millionaire Howard Hughes filed a lawsuit against TWA airlines—which had sued *him* just six months prior for allegedly violating antitrust laws. And sharing space with those stories on the front page of the *New York Times* business section that day was the following headline: "Kennedy Praised by Clothiers for Spurring Interest in Style."

The story chronicled the fourth annual press preview of the American Institute of Men's and Boys' Wear in 1962. There, clothiers from all over hailed President John F. Kennedy as "the most powerful and constructive influence on the manner and style of male attire."

More than 30 years later, nostalgia for the Kennedy style continues to exert a strong hold on the American imagination. Those were heady days for a young and optimistic nation, viewed through the mists of nostalgia as our own Camelot, when Jack and his wife, Jackie, entertained poets and politicians at elegant state dinners in the White House that were the envy of the world. It was as close to royalty as we've ever come. Or are ever likely to.

In Kennedy's brief but exalted life, he recorded what seems like several lifetimes' worth of accomplishments: He turned his senior thesis into a best-selling book in college. He served in the Navy during World War II, survived a harrowing Japanese attack, led his men to safety, and won Navy and Marine medals of heroism. He was a foreign correspondent and journalist. He won the Pulitzer Prize. He was the youngest man and the first Roman Catholic

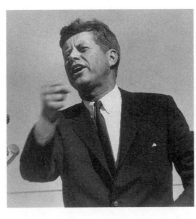

ever elected president. He fought arduously for and made monumental gains in promoting equality and smoothing race relations. He created the Peace Corps.

Kennedy's clothing contributions were memorable as well. As the *New York Times* chronicled at the time, Kennedy helped set the fashion standard. "The President is creating a handsome and responsible image of the American man," commented women's fashion designer Lilly Daché at the time. In a description that remains every bit as true today as it was at the time, Daché said that the ideal men's clothing look combines "Italian flair, classic British sobriety, and American dash, functionalism, and fit.

"In our president, we have the man who fits this look perfectly," Daché said.

"President Kennedy had immense influence on clothing styles, but there's still a lot that we don't know because he was such a private person," says June Payne, a reference librarian at the John Fitzgerald Kennedy Library in Boston.

"We may not know what he had in his pockets, what he used for shampoo or deodorant, or what he was feeling on the inside. But we know that on the outside he generally wasn't too concerned with keeping up the current men's fashion trends," Payne says. "We know that he liked single-breasted two-button suits, instead of three-button suits, and we know that he didn't wear a hat as often as other men."

Other fashion quirks that Kennedy was noted for include his reluctance to wear a topcoat. His tendency to carry his hat, when he had one, rather than wear it. His tendency to not hide the fact that he was wearing a belt rather than suspenders. He's also credited with helping repopularize the suit as standard daytime wear.

John F. Kennedy was assassinated on November 22, 1963 in Dallas. He was 46.

Miles Davis

The Birth of Cool

In the world of jazz, there was no one like him before and no one like him since.

Miles Davis exuded style, from his ever-evolving music to his trend-setting wardrobe, from his self-absorbed stage manner to the reck-lessness of his personal life.

Miles Davis and his trumpet first made their mark by helping to shape bebop jazz in the 1940s. Any musician would be proud to have set one new paradigm; Miles set new ones every few years, constantly inventing new jazz styles. The cool. Fusion. Modern. Where Miles went, other jazz musicians soon followed. Through a recording career that spanned nearly 50 years until his death in 1991, Miles never stopped creating new jazz forms.

Not that Miles was a saint. He was addicted to drugs twice—first, to heroin in the 1950s, then to cocaine in the 1970s. He could be cruel, even violent, to women. He was rude to his fans and fellow musicians. But ultimately, his musical genius and his hipness always tran-scended it all, and it is what will be remembered best about him.

"From the start, Miles had a certain aura of class," says Dan Morgenstern, former editor of the jazz magazine *Down Beat* and now director of the Rutgers University Institute of Jazz Studies in Newark, New Jersey, which holds the world's largest archive of jazz materials. Morgenstern had the good fortune of interviewing and spending time with Davis through the years. "He liked fast cars, good-looking women, and clothes. He was an extremely handsome man, very photogenic."

Esquire magazine once included him in a list of best-dressed men.

It was not his sharp blue suits, of course, but what he did with a blue note that qualifies

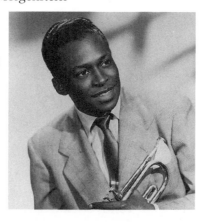

him as a man of timeless style.

At a time when jazz musicians were playing as many notes as they could, often as fast as they could, a Miles Davis solo was marked by how few notes were played. But what notes they were.

"The sound of Miles Davis is the sound of sadness and resignation," Joachim Berendt, an internationally recognized European jazz producer and authority, wrote in *The Jazz Book*.

Be it music, clothing, or political stance, Davis was always true to himself. He always did exactly what he wanted to do, without compro-mise. And sometimes it wasn't pretty. Davis turning his back on the audience, never introducing songs. Davis saying cruel things about other musicians. Davis being rude to fans. Davis being bigoted.

"I interviewed Dizzy Gillespie once, and he told me that Davis cultivated that image of someone hard to approach because he was a basically shy person," Morgenstern says. "I remember standing with Davis once at the Plugged Nickel, a club on Rush Street in Chicago, and some hapless fan approached him at the bar asking some inane question. Davis belched in his face."

His own distinctive voice, soft and raspy, was actually the result of his impatience. Following surgery on his vocal cords, doctors told him not to raise his voice. That was not Davis's style. He did and his voice was permanently impaired.

Despite his impatience and rudeness, "he really could be a very nice person, generous and pleasant," Morgenstern says. That view is borne out by the fact that he drew people so easily to him.

"He was a tremendous talent spotter," adds Morgenstern. "He knew how to surround himself with gifted people."

That, too, is the mark of a stylish man.

The Duke of Windsor

The King of Style

He was one of the most fastidious and fashion-conscious monarchs to mount the throne. Officially Britain's Edward VIII, the world knew him as the Duke of Windsor. Although he only held the crown for 325 days before voluntarily giving it up for the woman that he loved, his contributions to style endure.

Born June 23, 1894, as Edward Albert Christian George Andrew Patrick David, Edward's grand influence on style began as early as the 1920s, when he was still the Prince of Wales. Blessed with a thin frame that lent it-self to a variety of clothing strategies, he often mixed his wardrobe, wore dissimilar combinations, and experimented with everything from fabric to colors to patterns to accessories. So much did he thumb his nose at conventional royal fashion that everywhere Edward went, his clothing set the very latest trend in menswear. Even comic strip character Dick Tracy's famous felt hat comes from an Edward-inspired snap-brim model.

"Let it not be assumed that clothes have ever been a fetish of mine. Rather have I become, by force of circumstance and upbringing, clothes-conscious," Edward wrote modestly in his autobiographical *Windsor Revisited.*

Edward's contributions to fashion range far and wide. Certainly, having a thin frame, virtually unlimited financial backing, and the best tailors in London helped. But his most powerful attribute was his passionate, pioneering spirit. He broke free of the stuffy, buttoned-down traditions of English royalty, while maintaining an appropriate look that best expressed his individuality.

Among Edward's most famous innovations was showy

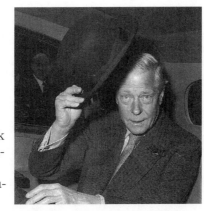

argyle socks worn conspicuously under golf outfits that were banded, rather than buckled, at the bottom. Another golf look debuted at Scotland's famed Saint Andrews course, where he topped off his outfit with a colorful Fair Isle sweater, sparking a run on similar garments so strong that, according to legend, it revived the area's flagging economy.

Formalwear, however, is where Edward excelled. Admitting a disdain for traditional formalwear, especially frock coats, Edward set a standard of easygoing elegance. His tailors made softer, pleated-front formal shirts with turned-down collars. He had his dinner jacket made in midnight blue rather than black because, he said, it looked "blacker than black" in artificial light. He also fashioned a double-breasted version, which became an instant hit.

In his life, Edward popularized suede chukka boots, Panama hats, snap-brim felt hats, raglan-style topcoats, and banded collars. He mixed plaids and checks, having personally inspired the dapper Prince of Wales check pattern. And, of course, he popularized—though he denied inventing it—the ubiquitous knot of choice for many men, the thick Windsor knot.

He spent his final days in France with his beloved wife, the twice-divorced American Wallis Simpson, writing, gardening, traveling, and tending his businesses. To the very end he held informal elegance and unaffected refinement in high esteem, even when it didn't concern clothing.

Near the very end, Edward suffered painfully through throat cancer. Less than two weeks before his death, he received a visit from his niece, the Queen; he insisted on dressing up for the occasion, even though it meant concealing the many tubes and fluid flasks attached to his body. Edward the Duke of Windsor died May 28, 1972.

Credits

Rodale Press gratefully acknowledges the following companies, shops, and people for providing the clothes presented in the book. Additional thanks to Dan Perio of Perio's Tailoring & Men's Shop in Bethlehem, Pennsylvania, and Mr. Frank A. Unger of Allentown, Pennsylvania.

Britches of Georgetowne, Herndon, Virginia

Suits:	page 82 (top and middle)
Jackets:	pages 85, 86 (middle and right)
Pants:	pages 90, 91
Overcoats:	pages 108 (left), 109
Shirts:	pages 98, 99 (top and middle)
Sweaters:	pages 104, 105 (top and middle)
Ties:	pages 86, 101

The Cedar Crest Stage Company, Allentown, Pennsylvania

Jacket:	page 86 (left)

Hartmarx: Consumer Apparel Products, New York, New York

Sweater:	page 105 (bottom)

The Legend Shoe Shop, Allentown, Pennsylvania

Shoes:	pages 118, 119

Leonard Logsdail, New York, New York

Suit:	page 82 (bottom)
Overcoat:	page 108 (right)

Worth & Worth, New York, New York

Hats:	pages 79, 80

Index

Underscored page references
indicate boxed text. **Boldface**
references indicate photographs.